C000146696

Table of Contents

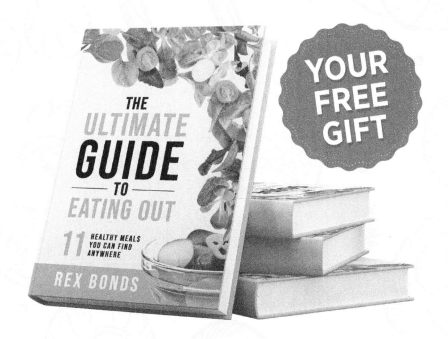

Before we get started, I'd like to offer you this free gift. It's my way of saying thank you for spending time with me in this book. Your gift is a Special Report titled, ***"The Ultimate Guide To Eating Out: 11 Healthy Meals You Can Find Anywhere."*** It's an easy-to-use guide that pulls together a ton of analysis I've previously only shared with clients. I think you're going to love it. This guide is a collection of 11 Healthy Meals you can find anywhere that will give you the system, tools, info, and mindset you need on the path to achieving your fitness dreams. This guide will teach you where to find clean, nutrition-packed meals to build lean muscle, burn fat and bump up your confidence in every situation no matter where you are.

**Scan Me
To Claim Your Free Gift!**

In this guide you'll learn:

✓ Where to find the 11 healthiest meals when you're eating out

✓ A rock-solid meal plan for any time of day & every location

✓ The exact script for which menu items to order

✓ Nutritional information for each dish at your fingertips

Plus as a Bonus!

✓ A Nutrition and fitness Journal to stay on track daily to your fitness dreams!

I'm willing to bet you'll find at least a few ideas, tools and meals covered in that guide that will surprise and help you. This guide will set you up for success and is a proven system when eating out. With this guide you will be armed with the info & focus you need. You will be giving your body nutritious fuel and enjoy eating out. With downloading this guide, you're taking a solid step on the path to your fitness success.

How can you obtain a copy of ***The Ultimate Guide To Eating Out: 11 Healthy Meals You Can Find Anywhere?*** It's simple. Visit RexBondsBooks.com and sign up for my email list (or simply click the link above). You'll receive immediate access to the Report in PDF format. You can read it online, download it or print it out. You will also get a Free Fitness Journal and Planner for signing up for my email list as well. Everything you need to get started and stay on your fitness journey is included in **signing up for my email list.**

Being on my email list also means you'll be the first to know when I release a new health and fitness book. I plan to release my books at a steep discount (or even free) for the first 24 hours. By signing up for my email list you'll get an early notification.

If you don't want to join my list, that's completely fine. This just means I need to earn your trust. With this in mind, I think you are going to love the information I've included in the ultimate guide. More specifically, I think you're going to love what it can do for your life.

Without further ado, let's jump into this book.

Join the Rex Bonds Fitness Community

Looking to build your specific fitness habits and goals? If so, then check out the Rex Bonds Fitness community: Rex Bonds Fitness Group

This is an amazing group full of like-minded individuals who focus on getting results with their lives. Here you can discover simple strategies, build powerful habits, find accountability partners and ask questions about your struggles. If you want to "level up" in your fitness journey, then this is the place to be.

**Just scan the QR code below
to join the Rex Bonds Fitness Community.**

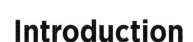

Introduction

Sugar sounds really pleasant these days, right? Eating a delicious pint of your favorite ice cream sounds pretty good right now, doesn't it?

But what do you do if you're the victim of obesity, hypertension, high cholesterol, diabetes, etc? Or better yet, what if these chronic diseases run in your family, and you fear ending up with them some day?

All of these problems have the same culprit: that sweet, sweet sugar.

Maybe you are aware that sugar is bad for your health. It actually can be the root cause of all your skin problems such as acne, rashes, eczema, dandruff; or even more serious problems like diabetes, high blood pressure, high cholesterol, obesity, and others. You may also experience that, even after taking regularly prescribed medications, these problems don't seem under control.

Why? Because you have not taken care of the primary cause: THE SUGAR.

However, it's easier said than done. Trust me, it's not that easy for anyone to ditch sugar completely. Maybe you are so obsessed with eating sugar, so heavily addicted to it that despite knowing it's bad effects, you can't control the urge. Each time your nose smells a sweet snack or your sight falls on it, you can't stop yourself from shoving it into your mouth.

Don't worry, it's not completely your fault. Going a day without sugar makes you feel weak, lethargic, angry, moody, and down. You might even feel bloated and anxious, maybe savoring those syrupy sweet snacks seems like a quick fix to your mood.

It could be that you want to get rid of your sugar cravings because you want to lose weight and shrug off all the health problems you are facing because of it; but the more you try to leave sugar, the more you crave it.

The solution? The 10-day sugar detox I will be unveiling in this book.

Here, I will guide you through the initial steps you should take to rid yourself of your sugar addiction in only 10 days. These initial 10 days are the toughest and I am here to help you in starting your "no sugar" journey.

Initially, you'll be eating no forms of processed sugars for 10 days, and then extend it to 30 days to see the full benefits it has on your health. Down the line, eating sugar-free food will become a part of your lifestyle and you won't go back to your old, unhealthy eating habits. That's a promise—genuine promise from Rex Bonds! I have trained hundreds of people to switch from a sugar-loaded diet to a sugar-free one and helped them achieve their health goals.

I understand the challenges many people face in going on a sugar-free diet. It makes them moody and angry. They never seem to feel full irrespective of the amount they eat from their plate. Their brain overpowers them to eat more, no matter how much they ate before. No logic, no reasoning can stop them from biting into any snack they can get their hands on.

I know that, like many of my clients, you may also face similar issues; and this is the exact reason I've written this book. I've done this to help you overcome your addiction to sugar, like I have helped many of my other clients.

And this is not just paying lip service to show off my success. I have a proof. One of my clients, Sarah, has been suffering from acne for the past 20 years. However, after the first week of sugar detoxing, she didn't feel like eating sugar anymore. The first week was like magic whereby I saw her skin clear up with no more acne. I call it magic because what 20 years of medical treatment couldn't do, one week of sugar detox did for her.

She was also overweight; but after, she felt healthier, didn't complain of bloating, could smell and taste better, and even lost 10 pounds of weight. No more lethargy, no anxiety, no depression, and she lost 5 more pounds after another 2 weeks of sugar detoxing.

Down the line after 3 months, she lost another 30 pounds of weight and living without sugar. All her other health problems disappeared, and she has the healthiest digestive system she has ever had in her entire life.

Another client of mine, David, dropped from 220 lb to 144 in less than a year; his blood pressure, blood sugar, and blood cholesterol levels returned to normal, and does need any of his medications now. The most powerful change was being in control of his food habits rather than allowing sugar and food controlling his life. He feels much better off without sugar and is mentally, physically, and emotionally stronger. David now tells me he craves for vegetables and proteins now instead of the donuts and ice cream from before the detox.

Although the results vary with every client, all of my clients are improving their relationship with food, have better immune health, spend less time in the doctor's office, genuinely feel good in their bodies, and are loving their bodies more and more each day. I know these results because many people have thanked me for how my training program changed their life for the better and changed their relationship with food to a far healthier one.

Now it's your turn to benefit from my training, which I'll reveal in this book. My training will equip you not only with physical results, but with the skills and knowledge to ditch your sugar addiction and be in complete control of what you eat.

Okay! So, now you know that you have me to help you with your sugar addiction, but what if you already feel healthy? Why would you need my training? Maybe you aren't ill or sick yet?

Don't wait till you get sick or have a health crisis to make healthier changes to your lifestyle. Start right now.

35% of the adult population in the United States has been diagnosed with pre-diabetic sugar levels. The life expectancy of children born after the year 2000 has declined. Why? Because of all the unhealthy sugary and fried foods kids are eating and exposed to nowadays. They don't have suitable role models whom they can look up to for leading a healthier lifestyle. Their parents suffer from chronic diseases due to an unhealthy lifestyle. Therefore, they follow the same lifestyle and are prone to suffer from chronic diseases.

Healthier people are more productive, spend less on healthcare, and have better job security. They are more active for home and social activities, spend less time in hospitals, doctor offices and pharmacies, have less pain and discomfort, and ultimately live a longer and better quality of life.

So, why miss out on the most valuable period of your life in disease? Why wait for your health?

You need to take action. Train your body and mind to live without the added sugars early and fast. Otherwise, you'll miss out on the most productive years of your life.

Luckily, you don't have to go far to learn these sugar detoxing tips. You have them right here! These proven methods yield results for people of all ages. Whether you are 20 or 40, these tips for detoxing sugar will be beneficial for you. Just follow these tips with perseverance.

In the initial four chapters, I'll be discussing the reason for your sugar addiction, our relationship with sugar as human beings, and then finally make you ready to ditch your addiction. Each following chapter will provide you with actionable steps to get rid of your sugar urges and make a permanent switch from unhealthy eating habits to a healthier controlled one.

So, let's start your sugar detox journey!

Chapter 01
The Drug That's 8x More Addictive Than Cocaine

Have you ever been told that sugar is 8x more addictive than cocaine? Well, what does it actually mean? Do you get hooked to sugar 8x faster than cocaine? Or are the withdrawal symptoms of sugar addiction are 8x worse than cocaine addiction?

Let's understand this with a popular research study.

In 2007, a study was conducted wherein rats were given two options: either consume a sweetened water solution or a cocaine water solution 8 times a day. 94% of the time, rats chose the sweetened water solution.

This study was further carried out in rats with cocaine addiction. Surprisingly, the researchers found that rats who were previously addicted to cocaine also chose the sweetened solution the majority of the time. This shows that sugar addiction develops so quickly and higher in rats that they forget about wanting the cocaine. They'll work much harder to get the sweetened water solution, even if they have to walk over a panel that repeatedly shocks them.

However, this was a study on rats. What about us human beings? Are we also addictive to sugar in a similar manner as rats?

The following example will make it clear on how sugar is addictive. But first, let us understand the difference between natural and refined substances.

There are substances that exist in nature without requiring much processing, such as tobacco leaves, beer from fermented barley, and sap from the opium plant. They become hazardous when you refine them far from their natural state. For example, tobacco is harmful to smoke in any form, but it takes frequent use over a lengthy period to reach that stage when smoked in its natural form. Similarly, the average person rarely drinks beer or wine to the point of addiction. Italian actor Dado Ruspoli smoked opium for 45 years without any severe implications on his health.

The bottom line? Substances become severely harmful and addictive ONLY when you refine them extensively.

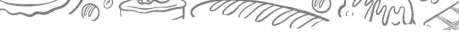

The Act of Refinement: Morphine, Cocaine, Alcohol

Around the year 1810, the substance morphine was derived from opium, and began use as a painkiller by American doctors in the 1850s—during the Civil war. Many injured soldiers were treated with morphine, and suddenly there were thousands of morphine addicts in the United States.

To tackle the situation, heroin was derived from morphine in 1874 and marketed as its non-addictive substitute. This is the main reason why heroin addiction is so prevalent in American culture.

Yet another example of this is cocaine addiction, which is also the product of refining the leaves of the coca plant. For ages, the farmers in the Andes Mountains chewed coca leaves for an energy boost. Though regular chewing was bad for their teeth, there was no other serious implication of chewing coca leaves because it was consumed in its natural state.

Even alcohol is not that bad unless you refine or distill it. You'll often see people ditch the beer and ciders and go for the hard liquor like gin, whisky, and vodka. People do this because you get more drunk on less alcohol. This is when you see people become really addicted to it and become alcoholics.

So, from these examples, we can see that the process of refinement makes a substance severely addictive. This happens because the refining process concentrates a particular ingredient in a given substance; like how cocaine concentration increases when you refine coca leaves or alcohol concentrates increases when you distill it.

So, when you consume the refined substance, it affects your brain's reward system and gives you a feeling of pleasure even higher than its natural counterpart. As the refinement process gets higher, the concentration of that ingredient increases and it has a larger effect on your brain's reward system.

This is because refined substances cause greater releases of dopamine in your brain, the hormone directly responsible for pleasurable feeling. Distilled alcohol makes you feel more drunk from less liquid. Cocaine and heroin make you feel even better from just a tiny bit of the substance. The effect is greater, even with a smaller quantity of the addictive substance.

How Sugar Affects Your Dopamine System

Now, let's come back to our addictive substance in question: THE SUGAR! Sugar is also the result of the refining process—specifically, refining the sugarcane. Refining concentrates a particular substance so much that the effects become even more intense. 100 kilograms of coca leaves when refined will give you 300-1200 grams of cocaine, and the resulting substance is 100 times stronger than what you started with. Similarly, for a good yielding sugarcane, half of the weight of one stalk is juice and 20% of that juice is sugar. There is not that much sugar in sugar cane because you have all that fibrous material that comes along with the juice. After refinement, the resulting substance will be 10 times sweeter than what you started with.

Compared to other tastes like salt or spice, sweetness activates your brain's reward system. Therefore, we are naturally programmed to seek out more sweet foods.

Another interesting fact about sugar is that it has a small, opiate-like effect. When doctors have to perform a circumcision of a newborn, they dip his pacifier in a sucrose solution called "sweet-ease", which is nothing but a concentrated sugar solution. This activates the brain's reward system of the baby, providing natural anesthesia to complete the procedure of circumcision without any fuss from the baby.

Do you know how much sugar an average American consumes in a day? It's nearly 82 grams or 26 teaspoons. So, let's do the math:

To naturally consume this much sugar, a person would have to chew around 2 pounds of sugarcane—in other words, 2 pounds of fiber-rich plant material. However, when you eat raw sugarcane, the fiber in the natural plant slows down the rate of which sugar releases into your system. But when you consume refined sugar devoid of fiber, it speeds up the rate of which sugar releases into your body.

A parallel way to understand this is cocaine. Your body can probably tolerate chewing through 100 grams of coca leaves because the active ingredient is released slowly. But what if your bloodstream is slammed with the active ingredient instantaneously? It will be a total shock to your body!

So, sugar has some parallels in other addictive drugs. But how is it addictive?

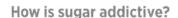

How is sugar addictive?

Sugar has been proven to be addictive to rats, as detailed in the study we discussed previously. However, to establish sugar addiction in humans, the criteria to classify a substance as addictive is a bit different.

According to the APA Diagnostics and Statistical Manual, any person should meet 3 out of 7 criteria to establish an addiction to an individual. These are:

1. Binging on the substance
2. Desire to quit using that substance
3. Craving or seeking the substance
4. Substance interfering with a person's daily life
5. Continuous use of the substance despite negative consequences
6. Tolerance to the substance
7. Presence of withdrawal symptoms

The first 5 criteria are psychological while the other two are physiological, which makes them the most important points to establish addiction in an individual.

It's easier to recognize "tolerance" objectively by using neuroimaging techniques. When you develop tolerance to a particular substance, the dopamine receptors in your brain get down-regulated. This means that more dopamine has to be released in order to have the same effect. As a result, you need more of that substance to get the same amount of pleasure.

Next, let's talk about "withdrawal". People who try to quit sugar often experience symptoms such as lightheadedness, headaches, anxiety, depression, mood swings, muscle aches, lethargy, fatigue, and physical tremors. In Morgan Spurlock's documentary *Supersize Me*, there is a section of the film where the actor says, "I was feeling bad in the car. Started eating, and now feeling crazy, feeling good." In essence, he was experiencing withdrawal symptoms which got better by eating again.

In the documentary, *That Sugar Film*, Australian Filmmaker Damon Gameau goes on an experimental high-sugar diet for 60 days. He consumed the same amount of calories every day, but only increased his sugar intake successively. In 30 days alone, he gained 8.5 kilograms or 19 pounds and by the 18th day; he had developed fatty liver disease. Finally, when he went off this diet, he experienced withdrawal symptoms, which he talks about in the film. *"Frankly, it didn't feel that much different from giving up cigarettes. I had headaches, I was moody, and my sleep patterns were terrible. I woke up very early and as soon as I was awake, I kind of felt like I'm craving sugar."*

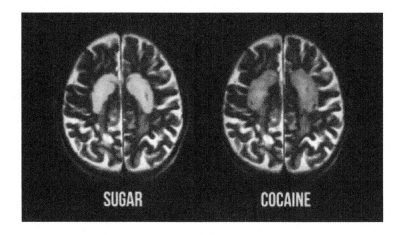

SUGAR | COCAINE

Evidence to Prove That Sugar is Addictive

Using the above MRI scans of a human brain, we can observe the sensory areas of the brain. The first person was given cocaine and the second was given sugar. You'll notice that the same sensory areas of the human brain light up in both persons.

So, what does that mean?

Essentially, it means that both sugar and cocaine affect the human brain in a similar manner. Since cocaine is addictive, so does sugar, which is proved by the MRI scans of the human brain above. Sugar is a food unlike the other highly-addictive substances we've discussed (cocaine, morphine, heroin, etc.); and yet, this experiment proves something different.

In the year 2007, another study was conducted on rats to prove the addictive potential of sugar. Rats were food deprived daily for 12 hours and then given a 12-hour access to the sugar solution after a delay of 4 hours in their normal daily eating cycle. The experiment continued for a month, and it was observed that rats learned to drink the sugar solution copiously, especially after the first access to it every day.

Moreover, these animals exhibited a series of behaviour similar to the effects of drug abuse. These behaviours included:

- Binging or large bouts of intake of the substance
- Withdrawal symptoms in the form of anxiety and depression
- Cravings for the substance high in sugar content
- Movement and eating behaviour similar to addiction by a drug substance

The Fastest & Easiest Way To Detox & Eliminate Sugar
In Only 10 Days To Lose Weight And Burn Fat

Thus, it was clear that sugar has the potential to create addiction similar to other drugs. So the question remained: "Why does this happen?"

This can be answered by looking at the brain images of these animal models. The addictive drug substances caused repeated, intermittent increase in the secretion of dopamine—the feel-good chemical—from the brain. Researchers found that rats with intermittent access to sugar drink the solution in a binge-like manner. This changes the expression of dopamine receptors in rats' brains.

Yet another explanation is that the rats with intermittent sugar access behave the same way as those with access to opiate drugs such as heroin, morphine, etc. Opiate drugs act on the brain by stimulating the release of dopamine and acetylcholine. Both of these effects are responsible for the withdrawal symptoms of opiate drugs.

The neurochemical adaptations of these rats' brains to intermittent sugar intake mimic the above effects of drug abuse, and thus, it can be formulated that intermittent, excessive intake of sugar has an addictive potential.

Therefore, although it is commonly available, refined sugar meets the criteria for the substance of abuse and can be "addictive" when consumed in a binge-like manner. This conclusion has been reinforced due to the changes in the brain that are similar for both drugs and sugar. Although the effects produced by sugar are smaller in magnitude than the drugs of abuse like cocaine and morphine, you can't deny the fact that they elicited the same effects by a natural substance like sugar.

The continual rise in obesity and these scientific findings establishing a parallel between hard drugs and sugar have given credibility to this idea. In a nutshell, it proves that sugar is addictive.

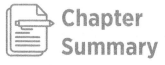 ## Chapter Summary

✓ Any substance—whether tobacco, alcohol, cocaine or sugar are harmful and addictive only—when they are refined extensively.

✓ The refinement process concentrates the particular ingredient in the substance, which is then released fast into the human body, thus creating its hazards.

✓ Sugar is as addictive as any other substance of abuse because it produces the similar effects on the brain as addictive drugs.

Chapter
02 The Last 1000 Years

The addictive potential of sugar has been validated, as we saw in the previous chapter. But one question remains: "Which is more addictive: Cocaine or Sugar?"

The majority of you will answer with, "Cocaine". That's because you think that giving up on foods like cakes, pastries, and sodas is far easier than a drug whose intake is also illegal. Well, you should give this a second thought.

Be it animals or human beings, we enjoy eating high calorie food more than anything else. The reason is simple: consuming high-calorie foods releases the feel-good chemicals like dopamine and endorphins in our brain, and obviously, we all want to feel good. The more we feel good the better right?

However, the problem is that it takes more and more of a stimulus to get the same amount of pleasure our bodies released the first time around. We need to consume high-calorie foods in ever-increasing amounts to get the same amount of pleasure from eating them every time. Thus, our cravings for high-calorie foods actually increase with every consumption.

Cravings have been there since the beginning of human evolution. Just go back to the ancient times and see what the ancient man ate. He hunted for the wild animals and ate their succulent and delicious flesh. That's because the cavemen had nothing else to eat right? No, they derived pleasure from eating it, and thus, craved for the same pleasure again and again.

However, imagine if their craving for the animal meat never returned! They would have died of hunger. Therefore, our brains were hard-wired from day one to crave substances that make us feel good, be it meat or refined sugar; and for a good reason. Food was scarce in ancient times, and anything high in calories like sugar or fat made sense to the caveman's brain. But these same pre-programmed actions of the brain confuse us today.

Today, we have sugar and refined carbohydrates in almost every food item, like bread, frozen ready-to-eat meals, candy, sodas, and pasta sauce. Our food choices have changed since the B.C. era, but our brains have not. Our brains still crave high-calorie foods. The problem is that they are everywhere now and readily available.

Imagine the situation if cocaine was just as easily accessible! Every other person would be seen consuming it, right? The same is happening with high-calorie foods like sugar. Since they are easily accessible now, their consumption has also increased. But these high-calorie and high-sugar foods mess with our hormones. The ancient cavemen had an eating schedule—they would either feast or starve. Unlike them, we are now constantly grazing on food, which makes our bodies and hormones go topsy-turvy.

Because we are consuming these high-calorie and sugar-filled foods, our bodies produce more insulin, which causes the energy from the food to be stored in our fat cells. Thus, overconsumption of high-calorie foods doesn't allow our bodies to burn fat. Thus, we are in the state of constantly storing it, thus becoming overweight and eventually obese as a result.

How to fix it?

Well, the only way to fix this problem is to cut down on processed foods. All processed foods have an ingredient list that doesn't contain natural items. Real foods don't have any such ingredient lists as they are the ingredients themselves. In simple terms, try eating like a caveman!

When you crave a snack, go for nuts instead of chips. For your sweet tooth, start consuming fruit over candy. Fruits are packed full of natural sugars as well as fiber that slows down the release of sugar into your bloodstream, thus keeping you full for a long time and curbing your in-between hunger pangs. Fruits are designed from the bottom up to have the perfect amount of fiber and sugar ratio that perfectly balances them out.

But do you know what the irony is? Every corner of the grocery store nowadays is loaded with chocolates, chips, and junk food. Even the stores that don't sell food items—like hardware stores, sports shops, and pharmacies—have junk food selections close to the register. Put simply, every time you visit a cash register, there's tempting junk food available at a relatively cheap price.

So, despite knowing those snacks are unhealthy, why are stores and supermarkets flooded with junk food? Because it sells. The junk food sells the most, and therefore stays on the market shelves while healthier things are more scarce and expire faster.

Food scientists are people who manufacture these processed foods in laboratories. They work with two simple goals in their mind:

- Make a product that will sell as much as possible
- Reduce the cost of production as much as possible

They are not concerned with making a product that is healthy for the consumers. How do they do this? Read on to know the answer!

Is low-fat also low in sugar?

Another buzzword that created a craze in the food industry in the 1990s was "low-fat", but it's time for a reality check.

Do you know why you are not losing weight despite switching over to low-fat or fat-free food items? Well, with many health-conscious consumers shifting towards low-fat foods, the food companies found another trick to lure you in, and sugar was their saving grace.

With the growing low-fat craze in the food industry, these companies were bound to make the food supply more and more overrun with added sugars. Because when you take out fat from a food item, you literally take out the taste from it. In order to counteract this effect, food companies add more and more sugar to the food items to make them appealing to your taste buds, while also maximizing their profits. As a result, you are still overdosing on sugar without really knowing it.

In fact, they understood that they can make anything taste better by adding sugar to it. Plus, they also know that sugar is addictive. That, and adding in excess sugar to "low-fat" and "sugar-free" foods is cheap and cuts down the cost of production.

Back in the 1300s, sugar was sold for 50 dollars a pound. But today, cultivation of sugarcane and beet sugar has improved considerably, and the refinement process has become much more advanced, cutting down the cost of sugar. Now a pound of sugar is roughly $2.50!

Moreover, with the invention of high fructose corn syrup, it becomes even cheaper. The United States produces massive amounts of corn and 32% of the world's corn supply comes from the United States. So, manufacturers were left over with a huge excess supply of corn but didn't know what to do with it; so they invented high fructose corn syrup. Using this addictive and economical substance in the food caused more and more people to buy it, because it is both identical to sugar and very cheap to manufacture. Simple business! Isn't it?

But the sugar they add isn't natural sugar—it's refined sugar.

There's another term in the "junk" food industry known as the "Bliss Point", which refers to the perfect amount of sugar, salt, and fat that optimizes an individual's palatability. In short, the amount of sugar, salt, and fat that should be added to any product to make you stuff more and more of it into your mouth.

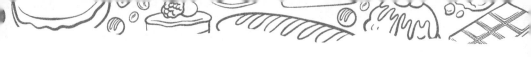

Suppose you are having a cup of coffee. If you keep adding sugar to it, it will get more and more delicious until you reach a point where it tastes too sweet. That perfect amount of sugar in your coffee cup is your bliss point.

Another term used in the "junk" food industry is "Mouth Feel". It involves studying the science of mouth feel to produce products that dissolve perfectly into your mouth. Food scientists study and manufacture such products to make them as satisfying as possible for the general masses while also leaving them wanting more. That's why those potato chips, for example, dissolve readily into your mouth, leaving you craving for more.

So, that's the reason supermarkets are flooded with junk food. The food has been engineered by the food scientists in a way to make it as irresistible as possible. Following the fabrication of these food items, you have the marketing that comes along with it.

These products are packaged in attention-grabbing colored bags with a variety of typography and child-friendly characters to grab your attention, especially to kids.

Besides, the most alluring and misleading of all marketing gimmicks are their health claims. They know that their consumers are becoming more health conscious. Therefore, they'll use buzzwords like protein, fat, cholesterol, gluten-free, etc. Let me warn you that you can disregard all these health claims as complete bullshit.

Take cereals or health bars as examples. Although they claim to be healthy, cereals are processed grains with sugar, salt, artificial flavors, and sweeteners. The same holds true for health bars, which are overloaded with hidden sugars. Other junk food can include yogurt, pasta sauce, bread, baked beans, soup, vitamin water, fruit juice, salad dressing, condiments, peanut butter, jam, chips, cookies, diet sodas and sports drinks.

All these products are packed with the same junk food formula of high amounts of sugar and salt. You may think you're eating healthy, but it's all a lie.

—————————— **"** ——————————

THE SIMPLE TRUTH IS THAT ALMOST ALL FOOD PRODUCTS ARE MADE WITH PROFIT MARGINS IN MIND AND NOT FOR THE CONSUMERS HEALTH.

—————————— **"** ——————————

Beware of Sugar on Your Food Labels

Okay! So, now you know that you were being duped by these food companies in the name of healthy food. What should the next step be if you really care for your health?

Well, ditch all those sugar-laden fat-free products from your kitchen shelves and make a healthy switch, of course!

But wait a moment! How will you recognize if a particular food item contains sugar or not? Sometimes you won't see "sugar" in the ingredients list when scanning the nutrition label. This is because food manufacturers are smart and figured out a way to disguise the sugar in your food as something else.

Sugar is known by a plethora of different names, making it easy for companies to hide how much sugar they add to the given product. Below, I have given you a whopping list of 56 different names for sugar! Some of them are obvious, while others are trickier to spot.

It may shock you to learn that over 68% of the bar-coded food items sold in the United States contain artificial sweeteners, even if the label says "natural" or "healthy". The US Foods and Drug Administration (FDA) has made it mandatory to display the nutrition label on all packaged food and beverages, including the sugar content per serving.

The best way to know if you are consuming added sugars or not is to get into the habit of scanning the ingredients list on your food products before dumping them into your shopping cart. Remember, ingredients are listed by quantity from high to low. So, the higher sugar is on the list, the more sugar present in that product.

Use this list of different sugar names to identify your addictive culprit.

The Most Common Names for Sugar (Excluding Artificial Sweeteners & Sugar Substitutes)

- **Basic Simple Sugars (monosaccharides and disaccharides):**

  - Dextrose
  - Fructose/Levulose
  - Galactose
  - Glucose
  - Lactose
  - Maltose
  - Sucrose

- **Solid or Granulated Sugars:**

  - Beet sugar
  - Brown sugar
  - Cane juice crystals
  - Cane sugar
  - Castor sugar
  - Coconut sugar
  - Confectioner's sugar (aka, powdered sugar)
  - Corn syrup solids
  - Crystalline fructose
  - Date sugar
  - Demerara sugar
  - Dextrin
  - Diastatic malt
  - Ethyl maltol
  - Florida crystals
  - Golden sugar
  - Glucose syrup solids
  - Grape sugar
  - Icing sugar
  - Maltodextrin
  - Muscovado sugar
  - Panela sugar
  - Raw sugar
  - Sugar (granulated or table)
  - Sucanat
  - Turbinado sugar
  - Yellow sugar

- **Liquid or Syrup Sugars:**

  - Agave Nectar/Syrup
  - Barley malt
  - Blackstrap molasses
  - Brown rice syrup
  - Buttered sugar/buttercream
  - Caramel
  - Carob syrup
  - Corn syrup
  - Evaporated cane juice
  - Fruit juice
  - Fruit juice concentrate
  - Golden syrup
  - High-Fructose Corn Syrup (HFCS)
  - Honey
  - Invert sugar
  - Malt syrup
  - Maple syrup
  - Molasses
  - Rice syrup
  - Refiner's syrup
  - Sorghum syrup
  - Treacle

So, don't let the food industry fool you in the name of low-fat or fat-free products. Low-fat products are actually high in sugar and calories and do more harm than good to your health.

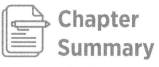

Chapter Summary

✓ Sugar is a high-calorie food and consuming such food releases feel-good chemicals (dopamine and endorphins) in our brain.

✓ However, the problem is that you need to consume sugar and other high-calorie foods in ever-increasing amounts to get the same amount of pleasure.

✓ High-calorie and high-sugar foods mess with our hormones.

✓ Frequent consumption of sugar and high-calorie foods results in increased production of insulin in our body, which causes the deposition of fat in the body cells.

- So, instead of burning fat, your body is in a state of constantly storing it, thus making you overweight and even obese.

✓ You might consume more than twice your daily recommended intake of sugar because of frequent consumption of packaged food and beverages.

✓ Sugar is a matter of disguise—it is known by at least 56 different names.

✓ Get into the habit of scanning the ingredients list of your food items and check for high sugar volume or added sugars before buying them.

Chapter 03
Deciding To Improve Your Health

By now, you must be motivated to switch to a healthier lifestyle and progress towards weight loss and better quality of life. Therefore, you can't miss this first step.

I know and understand your eagerness to jump into the list of foods to eat and create a new lifestyle of eating and nutrition. However, it's impossible to do so without deciding to do what is necessary to make that change first.

Taking this leap into a healthier life means that you are making a definitive choice. So, before we move ahead, make a decision—a decision to implement all the steps given in this book for your health, because it is worth it.

Well, making a decision is not difficult, but sticking to it is. That's because our bodies betray our mental commitment for our food choices. Therefore, I'll explain how sugar addiction affects our bodies physically further in the book to prepare you mentally and help you stay strong on your decision.

I'll walk you through step-by-step instructions on how to stop the cravings for high-sugar and high-calorie foods, as well as unwanted symptoms associated with such a diet. Once you gain the knowledge and understanding of which types of foods to avoid and the reason behind it, it gets a lot easier to make the right decision for your health and stick to it. You'll be able to take the next step, and then the next until you completely transform your lifestyle—a lifestyle that excludes chronic diseases and unwanted symptoms from your life.

The earlier chapters have proved the addictive nature of sugar due to the release of dopamine in our brains, thus augmenting our craving for carbs and sugary foods—refined carbs to be specific.

Refined carbohydrates include rice, wheat, white bread, cereals, potato chips, sodas, crackers, etc. Overconsumption of these refined carbs rewires our brain and nervous system, resulting in our addiction to them. As a result, despite negative consequences like weight gain and other health issues, people still binge on these types of food.

So, getting off sugar is more complex than it appears. It not only takes willpower and self-discipline, but you have to tackle the biochemical addiction. Thankfully, by implementing the steps given in this book, you can undo your brain's rewiring.

We live in a world today where we feel the need to satisfy ourselves to the heart's content. Moreover, delicious, unhealthy, sugary foods are available at our fingertips. You can even order them with just a click. In addition, TV commercials entice you to indulge and binge on such foods, which can also lead to addiction.

However, when you are addicted to something, you don't understand the concept of moderation (what the moderate quantity to consume is). In short, it's not feasible to just rely on moderation. What is required is an understanding of the causes that lead to the consumption of these foods in a manner you might not want to hear.

Are you attracted by the enticing bags and packages used for their marketing? Or are these foods inexpensive, quick, and easy to prepare? What makes you satisfy your immediate cravings with these foods without thinking about their long-term consequences on your health?

If you look at their actual cost, they seem inexpensive at the moment. In time, however, their ill-effects will show up in chronically poor health, increased medical costs, and the cost of pharmaceuticals to combat their effects. On the other hand, eating nutritious food prevents and even reverses the conditions better than the expensive medications.

Over 100 million Americans suffer from chronic, painful, and expensive disease conditions. The primary reason? Poor food quality! It's not that they are poor and can't afford high-quality products. The food industry wants them to eat their products; not for their health, but to fill their bank accounts. They understand human psychology and the addictive nature of sugar. So, if they use more sugar in their products, more people will buy them and return them the profits.

It's not that these Americans don't feed themselves with the proper nutrients they need to repair their bodies and reverse many of the chronic diseases they face. However, many of them are tired, have a foggy mind, or are too ill to make the right decision.

To improve the way you feel, you must stop eating sugar and refined carbohydrates. You have to make this decision. If you stick to this lifestyle, you'll lose weight and improve your health tenfold.

The problem is that most people don't take the step to improve their health until there's a crisis that forces them to make the change.

Many of my clients have gone through a health crisis, but one client in particular comes to mind. Her name is Sarah. She went through 20 years of medical treatments for her acne and eczema without an expected result. She had to either stay on

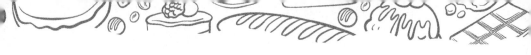

medication for the rest of her life or find an alternative.

So, she finally decided to do some research on her own. She discovered that sugary foods might be the culprit of her skin problems. She took a look at her own diet, which consisted mostly of sugary foods and refined carbohydrates. She decided to make a change and cut out sugar from her diet completely.

Can you guess what happened?

After a week, she didn't even want sugar and felt sick at the idea of turning back. Her skin cleared like magic, her acne healed completely, and she had a far more radiant skin than before. She also noticed the disappearance of her dandruff, which never returned. She was no longer out of breath going upstairs, felt healthier, could smell and taste things better, her belly bloating was gone, and she lost 10 pounds. She was also no longer depressed and lethargic.

Another client of mine, Rasheed, was 220 pounds, prediabetic, had high blood pressure despite taking medications, and had a crippling anxiety which he was also taking medication for. Tired of all his problems, Rasheed started taking action towards improving his health. That action was exercising and taking care of his diet.

I gave him a basic exercise program, and strictly told him to avoid any high-processed foods, refined carbohydrates, and sugary foods. Although it was hard in the beginning, Rasheed saw incredible results and stuck to the regime.

After three months of following my guidance to the letter, he lost 30 pounds and most of his chronic diseases went away. He was prediabetic, but no more. The inflammation of his body reduced drastically, and he was far happier as a result. He tried eating sugary foods, but they all seemed way too sweet once he cut them out.

In five months, he lost over 40 pounds. He started his journey in August when he weighed 220 pounds; but by January, he went down to 173 pounds. His jean's size was reduced from 38 to 32. His anxiety was gone and he felt more balanced, more positive, and had the best functioning digestive system ever. In less than a year, he dropped his weight down to 144 pounds. His blood pressure is perfect and under control without any medications. His triglycerides, cholesterol, and blood sugars are normal.

The most powerful change he noticed in himself is finally being in control of his diet, appetite, and food choices. Now, he has a much different and healthier relationship with food than before. It was hard to stick to a healthy diet when you are off sugar, but now he craves veggies and complete proteins.

Sarah, Rasheed, and many of my other clients agree that diet change requires an impressive deal of self-control. Still, they were determined to succeed and achieved their goal because they desperately wanted their health back.

These clients fought a war against their addiction, but you need not wait until something catastrophic happens to you, like landing with some chronic health issue. You can start right now, and I guarantee that once you regain control over your food choices, you'll see the benefits and all your hard work pay off.

Don't take your health for granted. Just like my clients, Sarah and Rasheed, who realized that their health is precious and learned they needed to take care of their health from now on.

So, ask yourself the following questions:

- Do you want your health back?
- Are you experiencing a health crisis and want a change?
- Are you overweight?
- Do you struggle with depression, mood swings, low energy, painful joints, diabetes, high blood pressure or any other health problem?
- Do you crave unhealthy and high-sugar foods?
- Do you need guidance on how to lose weight and improve your health?

If you answer "Yes" to any of these questions and really want to make a change, this book will provide you with step-by-step guidance and walk you through the process of regaining your health! It will provide you the blueprints you need to change your lifestyle for the better.

Let's start with the first step!

The first STEP to get off sugar and refined carbohydrates is to DECIDE. Decide to make the necessary changes and modifications. And it's ONLY YOU who can make this decision, no one else, because it's your choice whether or not you want to lead a healthy life.

However, your decision is your commitment. The subsequent chapters will help you maintain and stick to this life changing and life-saving decision. This book will also provide you with a support system, the right information, and the will to throw away all that junk from your house. Once you decide to change your lifestyle, you'll not only benefit yourself, but your family as well.

A diet high in sugar is also linked to Alzheimer's and dementia. Alzheimer's is a progressive brain disorder that causes the brain cells to waste away and die. It's one of the leading causes of dementia—a continuous decline in thinking, behavioral, and social skills that disrupt a person's ability to function independently.

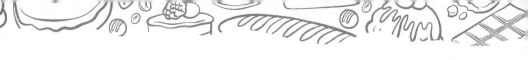

So, you need to start early before any symptoms of Alzheimer's or dementia appear.

Make your Commitment

Now that you have decided to take the step to improve your health and quality of life, follow the steps below that will help you stay accountable as well as give you measurements to track your progress along the journey.

- **Brain Testing:** Since you know now that the food we eat affects the function of our brain, start by taking this online cognitive test to determine the health of your brain. This online cognitive test helps you see where you are right now. The test is called Self-Administered Gerocognitive Exam (SAGE), at elderguru.com. Click on SAGE Alzheimer's Exam in the right lower panel.

- Next, write down your results from the cognitive assessment.

  _____

  _____

- Write a contract to yourself in the following format. Include the measurable goals you would like to achieve and sign it.

  I ___(name)_____ commit to eating no sugar and carbs for _ (number)_____ days.

  The results I want to achieve are

  _____

- **Baseline Assessment:** After deciding to get rid of sugars and refined carbs, you need to take certain measures before moving ahead. Before changing your lifestyle and eating habits, you need a baseline of your current position. Weigh yourself and measure your waistline.

- Jot down the following information:

  - **Date to Implement Changes:**
  - **Baseline Measurement Date:**
  - **Weight:**
  - **Waistline:**

- **Symptom Checklist:** Put a check next to all the symptoms you have or experience currently:

  ☐ Anxiety

  ☐ Chronic Fatigue

  ☐ Fibromyalgia characterized by musculoskeletal pains, fatigue, sleep, memory, and mood issues

  ☐ Decreased Sex Drive

  ☐ Depression

  ☐ Foggy brain

  ☐ Food allergies

  ☐ Insomnia/ inability to sleep

  ☐ Irritability

  ☐ Hormonal imbalance

  ☐ Poor memory

  ☐ Craving sweets and refined carbohydrates or alcohol

  ☐ Digestive problems like constipation, diarrhoea, or bloating

  ☐ Skin and nail infections like toenail fungus, athlete's foot, and ringworm

  ☐ Vaginal yeast infections

  ☐ Urinary tract infections

- **Dietary Assessment:** Record all the of foods you ate in the past week. Mention if sugary foods, processed foods, and refined carbohydrates are an enormous part of your diet. This is so you have an understanding where your diet is at currently.

  Day 1 _____

  Day 2 _____

  Day 3 _____

  Day 4 _____

  Day 5 _____

  Day 6 _____

  Day 7 _____

The Fastest & Easiest Way To Detox & Eliminate Sugar
In Only 10 Days To Lose Weight And Burn Fat

After these initial steps, you are ready to take on the journey for the next 10 days. These first ten days will be the toughest. But after 30 days, and after 6 months, you'll start seeing the best results.

After 6 months of changing your eating habits, measure your cognitive abilities again—this includes your weight, waistline, and whether or not any unhealthy symptoms subsided.

Chapter Summary

✓ The first step to getting off sugar and refined carbohydrates and switching to healthy eating habits is to DECIDE to make that change.

✓ However, sticking to your decision is tough because it takes a great deal of willpower, self-discipline, and tackling your biochemical addiction to sugar.

✓ It gets a lot easier if you follow the steps outlined in this book with perseverance.

• Don't wait for any health crisis to crop us to switch to healthy eating habits. Decide right now for your health.

✓ Once you decide to make the transformation, follow the steps given in this chapter to note down your baseline measurements. This keeps you accountable and makes it easier to track your progress.

The Knowledge and Support System For Success

The next step after deciding to make the change is to build your support system. But what is that exactly, why do you need it, and how do you build one?

Let's answer these questions in this chapter!

Importance of Developing a Support System

You will experience ups and downs along this journey of health. It's natural. Therefore, you need people who can understand you and are dependable during the tough times. People who will listen to you and give honest feedback. Such people form your support system and give you benefits such as:

★ **Higher levels of well-being**

★ **Better coping skills**

★ **Longer and healthier life**

Studies can attest to the need for a support system in decreasing stress, depression, and anxiety. In fact, giving and receiving support from others is a basic human need.

So, if you want to bring your grim mood up and stay on the path of achieving your health goals, you need to develop a support system—a system consisting of people you can trust and who will keep you accountable.

To build such a network, start with the people already in your life. Make a list of these people. From there, determine who is a healthy and positive influence and who is not. Then, limit the contact with negative people in your life, especially when you are on this health journey. That's because these negative people will drain your energy and bring you down. Making a list of the positive people already in your life is beneficial, and listing the negative people will open your eyes to those you don't really want in your life.

Use this table to list the names of positive and negative people in your life:

+ Positive People	− Negative People
_____	_____
_____	_____
_____	_____
_____	_____
_____	_____
_____	_____
_____	_____

Making changes to adopt a different lifestyle demands energy. Therefore, you need people who support you and have your back 110%. Your time and energy should be invested in those who make you feel good about yourself, and not have the opposite effect. Therefore, watch out for any such negative people around you: blamers, liars, alcoholics, drug abusers, and those who put you down.

Your support network can have people from:

Family

Friends

Neighbors

Office

Gym

Social Media

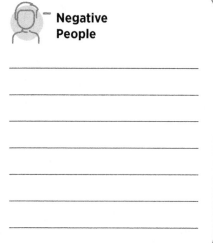

Mental health professional(s)

Support groups that have people experiencing a similar situation

Support group websites

Here are some helpful tips for building your network of positive and supporting people:

1. Review your current family and friends; evaluate who can be helpful.
2. Try new activities to engage with new people.
3. Join a book club.
4. Be a member of any sports team.
5. Let important people in your life know that you appreciate them.
6. Willingly ask for help when needed.

Four Simple Strategies to Achieving your Health Goals

Research proves that people who set goals are successful, but only 8% of them actually achieve their goals. Here are some proven strategies to increase your chance of achieving your health goals:

1. Find a support system.

Your environment and social surroundings play a great role in whether or not you'll achieve your health goals.

Just think! If you are surrounded by people eating donuts and candy every day, how can you expect yourself to not crave and/or eat sugar? The simple solution is to get a support system where you'll have people sharing your vision and keeping you accountable. This support system will also help you focus on your goals. Also, your environment matters. If you hang out with people who eat candy and donuts every day, then you are way more likely to do that yourself.

2. Have a purpose behind your goal.

Why do you want to lose weight? Why do you want to achieve your goals?

In short, setting a goal should have a purpose. Don't set it just for the sake of setting a goal. Otherwise, you are more likely to fail when faced with challenges. When you have a purpose behind your health goals, and even write them down, you ease your path to success. They become a tangible driving force to reach the target.

For example, you might wish to lose weight to fit in that wedding dress. Or you wish to join a marathon this year, and therefore build endurance by exercising more. Whatever your purpose, it motivates you to keep pushing when the going gets tough.

3. Create smaller goals that build up to your ultimate goal.

There's a saying, "You should set SMART goals". SMART stands for Specific, Measurable, Achievable, Relevant and Time-bound. Keeping this in mind, you set a goal to lose 30 pounds by the end of the year. Now, that's SMART, but there's a problem.

Big goals are daunting and can make you feel overwhelmed. However, when you break them down into smaller milestones, they are less intimidating and will keep your focus on track. When you achieve those smaller milestones, you automatically build courage to achieve the bigger ones. An example would be if you want to lose 30 pounds by the end of the year, then you would want to lose just 2.5 pounds a month and just a little more than ½ a pound a week! See? It's not so much of an intimidating daunting task when you break it down!

4. Reward yourself.

Every achievement calls for a celebration! When you see progress in your health goals, take pride in yourself. Reward yourself with something you always wanted, even at smaller achievements, and don't wait until the end. This boosts your morale and brings positive reinforcement towards your health goals.

Finally, the consistency that pays off, be it your health goals or any other goal in life. Implement these strategies regularly and get ready to welcome the new you.

Let's face it! It won't be easy to stay motivated for every meal and workout on this health journey. From early morning wake-ups to healthy diet choices, switching to a healthy lifestyle takes serious mental grit. Ultimately, it's your willpower that will lead to success. You need not set off on this journey alone. Building and fostering a strong supportive community of family, friends, and fellow health enthusiasts will keep you motivated and stay on track when things seem hard.

Now, we'll take on some top questions beginners have on this health journey.

How important it is to have a strong support system when beginning my no sugar journey?

It's extremely important to have at least one person as your accountability partner in your journey. They can be a friend, spouse, co-worker, training partner, personal trainer, or anybody on the same mission as you. We suggest choosing a person who is willing to go on a no sugar diet with you or has already gone through it. They might be willing to go on walks with you. This way you can call, email, or connect and tell each other what you ate throughout the day. You can also send pictures to each other and keep one another accountable.

How can a supportive community help me reach my health goals?

Along this journey, you'll encounter times when you don't feel like eating healthy or have sugar cravings. That's where the role of the supportive community sets in. If you have a supportive and dependable person in your life, they can help you overcome these challenges and get you on track. In case you end up eating unhealthy food on a given day, they can call you out on it and make you aware of what you need to do to get back on track.

What if someone I know and trust opposes my transformation and/ or goals? What if it is my spouse or family member? How do I stay on track and push ahead?

Surprisingly, this is very common. Many people go through this all the time. You might deal with people who want to get revenge on others who criticized or mocked them for not looking their best. It's called a "revenge body".

A couple I worked with comes to mind. The wife really wanted to lose weight, but the husband was reluctant. He felt threatened that if his wife lost weight, she'd look better than him and might even leave him.

It's important to have a conversation with the people who want to sabotage you. Explain to them the importance of this journey for you. Ask them clearly to help you with your journey or else stay out of your way. If they still try to undermine you, steer clear of them and focus on your goals.

If I am going solo, how do I build a community from scratch?

Some of you might be in this position, but there has to be at least one person in your life. It might require you to approach someone new, like a coworker, a loved one, or finding groups on Facebook and other social media.

What kind of people are important to have in my circle?

Basically, the supportive ones who motivate you when going gets tough and keep you accountable.

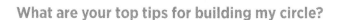

What are your top tips for building my circle?

Start where you are and with people you know. Besides, we are all building communities right here and right now. At Rex Bonds Books, we are literally creating communities of fitness enthusiasts and anyone interested in health who are coming together with common goals, interests, and curiosity to find new ways to enjoy physical exercise, diet, and fall in love with their health. You can find this group here: https://www.facebook.com/groups/541464226513612/edit/

What about people who are introverted or shy? Do they have a harder time building a community? What would you advise them?

Yes, sometimes these people find it hard to build a supportive community. However, they can look for someone similar to themselves through apps or on our Facebook group.

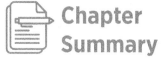

Chapter Summary

✓ It's important to have a support group or community on this journey to health and quitting sugar.

✓ A supportive community keeps you on track, accountable, better coping skills, and gives you a higher sense of well-being.

✓ Your support group will also decrease your stress, depression, and anxiety.

✓ Your supportive community can be composed of people from your family, friends, neighbors, gym, social media, or anyone who shares the same health goals as you and is ready to give their 110% back to you in tough times.

✓ To build your supporting network of people, start with where you are and who is in your life. Keep the ones who are positive about their health and eating habits while limiting contact with negative people.

Chapter
05 Clean Out Your House

You have decided to change your eating habits and build your support system as well. Now it's time to clean out your house, pantry, and refrigerator of all unhealthy and unwanted food. This is a crucial step to help you keep away from the temptations of eating such food items.

I know it's tough, but you might need to use your support system here for willpower and accountability to take actions in this step.

Why do you have to remove all unhealthy food?

Food triggers like cookies and ice-cream can cause you to relapse into your old eating habits. By simply looking at these food items, dopamine is released and causes an overwhelming desire to consume them. Therefore, it's necessary that you get rid of them.

However, another challenge is having a family member who wants to consume these foods. This may tempt you to eat them as well, but there's a solution! Tell them to keep these packages hidden in their room and out of the pantry or refrigerator. Ask them kindly to honor your goals and help you along your journey.

I like to classify foods as either "dead" or "alive". A food item that's been sitting on the shelves in the store for months is dead. It won't give your body the nutrients it needs to be healthy. On the other hand, a fruit or vegetable needs to grow and contains essential vitamins, minerals, nutrients, and fiber required by your body. The fiber in fruits and vegetables fills your stomach and signals your body when it is full. Furthermore, the fiber slows down the digestion and release of sugar in your body, thus preventing a sudden rapid sugar surge in your blood.

This fiber gets removed in processed foods, so you need a larger quantity to become full.

When you eliminate these unhealthy processed foods from your diet, you'll be munching on whole organic fruits, vegetables, whole grains such as oats, brown rice, quinoa, barley, beans, fish and meat.

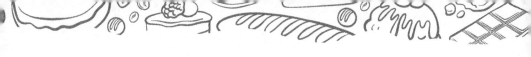

Foods to Eliminate from Your Diet

Understanding what types of food are harmful versus what types are beneficial is confusing today. The food industry does an excellent job of enticing us through addictive ingredients and their marketing tactics.

First, check the food labels of your items when you go grocery shopping, and do not buy products with more than 5 ingredients or 10 grams of sugar per serving. If you encounter an ingredient you can't pronounce, then your body probably won't recognize it well.

If you are really unsure about the product, it is better not to buy it. Eating fresh fruits, vegetables, and meat will ultimately cost you less and will be better for your health.

Here's the list of food items to eliminate from your diet:

Wheat

I do not recommend eating any food containing wheat because nowadays wheat is hybridized. This means it is not the same grain that has been used throughout the centuries. Today's wheat is extremely hard to digest, and this is why we see an increase in the number of gluten sensitivity cases.

White Flour

White flour is one of the most common and prevalent wheat products used today. However, the fiber and nutrients in white flour are chemically bleached. Since the revolution of grain milling, it's easy to separate the components of the wheat berry. This removes the fiber and nutrients significantly and extends the shelf life of white flour.

If any nutrients and natural oils are left in the flour, they would become rancid after sitting some time on the shelf, but the food industry is smart. It prefers products with a longer shelf life so their products will not go bad sitting on the shelves and can be sold for longer periods of time. Products made from white flour have no nutritional value.

Sugar and High Fructose Corn Syrup

White Rice

White rice is also similarly processed as white flour. To extend its shelf life, the husk, bran, and germ are removed, thus removing the grain's nutrients. Instead, consume brown rice and wild rice, as they contain all the fiber and nutrients in them.

Corn

Most of the corn in the United States has been genetically modified to make it resistant to insects or herbicides. Consequently, farmers spray as much insecticide on corn as necessary. Also, your body can't digest corn well, so bid goodbye to popcorn and tortilla chips.

Limit the Consumption of Milk Products

A nutritional source of Calcium, protein, and minerals, today's milk is also stripped of its nutritional value to extend its shelf life.

Food industries heat raw milk to high temperatures (pasteurization), which destroys all the microorganisms and most nutrients. So, they add vitamin D to milk to counteract this effect. Raw milk contains enzymes that help with digestion, but they are lost after pasteurization. This is why lactose intolerance is so high today.

Also, humans are the only mammals on earth that still drink milk after the age of 2. This milk is supposed to help a baby calf grow 4x its size in only two years. Moreover, we don't drink milk from a human, but from a cow. If you stop consuming dairy products, you will naturally lose weight.

Instead, consume almond, cashew, or coconut milk products and kefir. Kefir is a fermented product that contains natural probiotics. Also, making your own almond milk is easy. The only ingredients you need are almonds and water. You will also need a blender and a cheesecloth to filter the milk from the almonds.

Soy Milk and Soy Products

Most of the soy crops in the United States are genetically modified. But if they are organic, it's healthy to consume.

Artificial Sweeteners

Artificial sweeteners are a strict no-no. People who frequently consume these sugar substitutes are at an increased risk of excessive weight gain, type 2 diabetes, and cardiovascular disease.

Moreover, sugar substitutes make you crave sweets. Artificial sweeteners are in many things, but the major culprits are diet sodas. Many people think they are consuming healthy food because that diet soda says 0 grams of sugar, but they are substituting the sugar for artificial sweeteners. And research proves that diet sodas make you crave more sugar and increase your body fat.

Dried Fruits

Dried fruits are packed with nutrients, but the drying process removes water and concentrates all the fruit sugar into a small bite, thus making them unhealthy and full of sugar. It also takes more dried fruit to fill you up compared to their whole fruit counterparts.

Dates and raisins are about 60-65 percent sugar. Dried figs are around 50 percent sugar. Prunes are about 38 percent sugar.

Processed Meats

Hot dogs, ham, bacon, sausage, and deli meats were classified by the World Health Organization as a group 1 carcinogens. This is the same class as tobacco, asbestos, and plutonium. Avoid purchasing any pre-packaged meats. You can instead bake a chicken or a turkey breast, cut it up, and enjoy it for lunch.

Vegetable Oils

Most vegetable oils contain omega-6 fatty acids which produce inflammation in the body. You want to decrease this and increase the Omega-3 fatty acids found in avocados, nuts, and fish. Omega-3 fatty acids also nourish your brain.

Extra virgin olive oil is the best and preferred oil for use. Extra virgin coconut oil and avocado oil are also great and can be used at higher temperatures because they resist oxidation at high heat.

Processed Foods

Have you ever noticed that all the fresh foods and ones you should eat are at the outside edges of the grocery stores? In the middle of the grocery store are the processed foods contained in boxes and bags. Do not eat any processed food that comes from a box or bag. These include cereals, chips, crackers, granola bars, cookies etc.

Peanuts

Contrary to the popular belief, peanuts are not a nut, but a type of vegetable called a legume. They grow from the ground and not a tree. Peanut butter is not recommended because it is hard to digest. Almond or cashew nuts are some of the better choices.

Margarine

Margarine mostly contains trans-fat which increases your risk of heart disease. Instead, use organic butter, olive oil, or coconut oil.

Canned Food

Canned foods are lined with BPA to prevent erosion of the can. Also, many preservatives are used in canned goods to increase its shelf life. Instead, go for fresh fruits, vegetables, and dried beans.

Microwavable Food

This can range from popcorn to frozen dinners. When you microwave food or beverages, the microwave heat alters the food, decreases the hemoglobin, and raises the bad cholesterol. I recommend reheating food in a toaster oven and limiting the use of your microwave.

Fruit Juice & Juice Drinks

Fruit juice contains lots of concentrated fructose and sugar, as they are devoid of fruit pulp and fiber. This is a direct invitation to obesity and diabetes.

Although juice is high in vitamins and antioxidants, you still should not drink any of it. Juice drinks, juice cocktails, and juice boxes are usually marketed for children and contain only 10% actual fruit juice. The rest is loaded with high fructose corn syrup or other sweeteners.

Diet Drinks

Even though diet drinks and sodas have zero calories and zero sugar, steer clear from these poisonous beverages. These artificial chemical sweeteners are heavily added to diet drinks. They are proven health hazards, as they stimulate your appetite. The caramel coloring added to these drinks is a known carcinogen, and the phosphoric acid in soda leaches calcium out of your bones.

Low-Fat Options

There was a huge fat-free food craze in the 1990s. Since fat-free foods were in-demand, food manufacturers added sugar and other flavorings to make up for the missing fat because it tasted so bad.

At that time, people did not think about the calories or sugar they consumed, their only focus was on the number of grams of fat they ate. Consequently, the average American has gone up 40 pounds since 1990, and obesity rates have doubled since then.

Dietary fat is important to host vital functions in your body, like producing hormones, conducting nerve impulses, absorbing certain vitamins, building cell membranes, and regulating your immune system. It also has the important job of breaking down carbohydrates, so you get a smaller insulin response

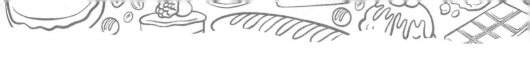

when you eat fat with your food.

Eating high carb and low-fat food increases the amount of insulin your body releases, leading to obesity and insulin resistance. Fat has more calories per gram than carbs or protein, so eating fat helps you feel full.

Diversely, eating low-fat, high-carb and high-sugar foods put your blood sugar levels on a roller coaster. Although not all fats are good fats, you need healthy monounsaturated fats from oils, fish, nuts, and seeds. Minimize the intake of unhealthy trans-fats from hydrogenated oils and saturated fats.

Getting into action to throw unhealthy food

Set a particular date in the month when you'll clean out your pantry and refrigerator of all the following food items:

- Any food item containing wheat
- Sugar-sweetened drinks like sodas, fruit juice, soft drinks
- White sugar, table sugar, high fructose corn syrup, or any type of syrup
- White rice
- Corn and corn products
- Artificial sweeteners like aspartame, saccharin, NutraSweet, sucralose, Splenda, maple syrup, agave, coconut sugar, monk fruit sugar, etc.
- Honey
- Hydrogenated oils
- Processed foods like chips, crackers, cookies, cereals
- Any food containing MSG
- Processes meats such as ham, bacon, sausage, hot dogs, lunch meat
- Margarine
- All milk products except Greek Yogurt with less than 5 grams of sugar per serving
- Packaged frozen meals
- Candy
- Baked treats like cakes, pies, Danishes, donuts, pastries etc.

After cleaning out, check all that applies:

➦ Did you clean out your pantry? **Yes/No**

➦ Did you clean out your refrigerator? **Yes/No**

➦ Did you clean out your freezer? **Yes/No**

Don't bang your head trying to decipher the food labels or count your sugar intake in grams. Make things simple for yourself. If it's not a plant, a protein, or a healthy fat, don't buy it for your family. If your daily meals are healthy and sugar-free, you need not fret when you're eating out on special occasions.

Chapter Summary

✓ The first step to changing your eating habits is to clean all of the unwanted and healthy food out of your house, pantry, and refrigerator. Instead, keep a stock of healthy food at home.

✓ It's vitally important that your kitchen or pantry is NOT loaded with junk and high-sugar foods, because your brain will drive you to eat them as they are more handy, and you'll relapse into your old eating habits.

✓ Eliminate these foods from your house, pantry, and refrigerator:

- Anything containing wheat
- Artificial sweeteners
- Aodas, fruit juice, & soft drinks
- Honey
- White sugar
- Any form of syrup
- White rice

- Corn products
- Limit dairy products
- Hydrogenated oils
- Processed foods
- Anything containing MSG
- Margarine
- Candy & baked treats

Chapter 06

Replacing The Junk

After cleaning out your home, pantry, and refrigerator of all unhealthy food, it's time to restock and purchase healthy food items you'll be consuming.

You won't be eating wheat, rice, processed foods, and anything with sugar; so what are you gonna eat now? Of course, it will be a complete change to your diet, and it might seem radical and limiting to you. Thankfully, you still have a plethora of options from different types of fruits, vegetables, and meats.

You can replace your ice cream or anything sweet with fruits, which can be thought of as nature's candy; but do so sparingly. Plus, you have access to different vegetables your body needs for various nutrients, proper growth, and performance.

Besides, you have grains as a source of carbohydrates such as amaranth, barley, buckwheat, millets, oats, quinoa, brown rice, rye, and wild rice. Nuts and seeds are excellent sources of protein and are recommended to be eaten raw without adding anything to them.

The plus with fruits and vegetables is that they are seasonal, so different types of fruits and vegetables are harvested at different times in the year. For example, strawberries ripen in the spring, okra and peas grow in summers, pumpkins mature in the fall, and so on. I always recommend eating fruits and vegetables of that season to derive maximum nutrition you need. Also, it will keep you from getting bored of the same type of food all year long.

Sometimes we get into the habit of eating the same type of food over and over again. But it's crucial that you eat an assortment of foods to get a variety of nutrients. And it's damn easy nowadays, since you can get hold of a variety of fruits, vegetables, grains, nuts, and seeds. You need to eat different types of food in these categories to take care of your body and function at your highest potential.

You can even buy a new fruit and vegetable every week at the grocery store. This will remove the fatigue of cooking the same meal over and over again. You may even find something that you love to eat by stepping out of your comfort zone.

What foods can you actually eat?

While on this no sugar diet, you can consume the following foods safely. In the later chapters, I've also added recipes to make it easier for you to eat sugar free. These foods are a step towards your no sugar journey:

All Meats

Beef, chicken, lamb, pork, turkey, bison, venison, duck. However, make sure these meats don't have added sauces or marinades to it. Purchase the freshest ones that only contain the meat of your choice. Always go for organic, grass-fed, or free-range with no hormones or antibiotics—these are the highest quality meats you can find.

All Seafood

Anchovy, bass, carp, catfish, char, cod, flounder, haddock, halibut, herring, mackerel, Mahi Mahi, sardines, salmon, trout, and tuna are the most popular types of fish on the market. Also crab, crayfish, lobster, prawns, shrimp, abalones, clams, mussels, oysters, octopus, scallops, sea snails, squid are all amazing options you can eat. Just like the meats, only purchase seafood with no added sauces or marinades.

All Vegetables

Artichoke, arugula, asparagus, avocados, green beans, bitter melon, bok choy, broccoli, brussel sprouts, cabbages, carrots, cauliflower, celery, collard greens, cucumber, daikon, eggplants, ginger, kale, leeks, lettuce, mushrooms, okra, onion, peas, peppers, pumpkin, radishes, shallots, squash, spinach, swiss chard, tomatoes, turnips, watercress, and zucchini are some of the many vegetables you can eat. You have many options here that you can enjoy and eat, but also many more to explore and try!

Low-Glycemic Fruits

Limes, strawberries, apricots, grapefruit, lemon, cantaloupe, guava, nectarines, oranges, pear, watermelon, blueberries, peaches, plums, apples, and kiwi are low-glycemic fruits. Low-glycemic fruits increase the blood sugar slowly and steadily, and are therefore the best to consume.

All Nuts & Seeds

Brazil nuts, almonds, pistachios, pine nuts, walnuts, pecans, hazelnuts, cashews, macadamia nut, sunflower seeds, pumpkin seeds, hemp seeds, chia seeds, flaxseeds and sesame seeds are all high-energy fuel sources packed with protein, fatty acids, vitamins, minerals, fiber, and other nutrients.

However, the nuts and seeds you consume should not be toasted, dry roasted, blanched, or salted. They should instead be minimally processed straight from the tree or plant they are derived from.

Legumes & Beans
Lentils, white beans, split peas, pinto beans, kidney beans, black beans, navy beans, lima beans, chickpeas, and mung beans are an inexpensive, heart-healthy food that is popular around the world. High in protein, legumes and beans are also good sources of iron, fiber, and potassium.

Whole Grains
Amaranth, barley, brown rice, buckwheat, bulgur, farro, millet, oats, quinoa, wild rice, rye, sorghum, spelt, and teff are all amazing whole grain options you can eat.

All Spices
Cumin, chili powder, paprika, nutmeg, ginger, oregano, garlic powder, turmeric, thyme, basil, cayenne pepper, bay leaf, saffron, curry powder, rosemary, onion powder, black pepper, sage, anise, coriander, cardamom, salt, crushed red pepper, smoked paprika, garlic, cinnamon, clove, and allspice are some of the best spices you can use to make your meat and vegetables taste amazing.

Beverages
You can consume sugar-free teas, unsweetened almond/nut milk, and water as daily beverages.

Condiments
Homemade hot sauce, coconut amino, apple cider vinegar, and red wine vinegar are some condiments you can use. For oils, use avocado, coconut, and olive oil for cooking.

Eggs & Butter
You can eat as many eggs as you want! Scrambled, poached, or boiled is up to you. You can also use butter to cook! The best and highest quality of butter is Kerrygold Butter. This butter is made from grass-fed cows and is healthy to consume.

Sugar-Free Protein Powder

Bob's Red Mill Protein & Fiber Nutritional Booster, Garden of Life Raw Organic Plant Protein Unflavored Powder, Nutiva Hemp Protein, Amazing Grass Protein SuperFood The Original, Vega One Organic All in One Shake Plain Unsweetened, Sunwarrior Protein Warrior Blend Natural, John's Killer Protein Grass-Fed Whey Isolate Protein, NorCal Organic Classic Whey Protein Concentrate, Vitals Protein Unflavored Collagen Peptides, PROMIX Micellar Casein Unflavored Protein Powder, and Designer Whey Natural 100% Whey Protein Concentrate and all amazing high quality protein powders with no or less than 1g of sugar in every serving of these specific protein powders.

Regardless of what you choose, unsweetened protein powder is a versatile staple in a healthy pantry. These protein powders are completely free of any sweeteners, including sugar, artificial sweeteners, non-nutritive sweeteners like stevia or monk fruit extract, and sugar alcohols.

It's always recommended to go for sugar-free protein powders because these protein powders are generally consumed by mixing with fruits or other ingredients that are naturally sweet.

Foods to limit or avoid eating altogether

Limit the consumption of the following:

- ☐ Monk fruit
- ☐ Stevia
- ☐ High glycemic fruits like cherries, mangoes, grapes, pineapples, prunes, watermelon, prunes

- ☐ Dark Chocolate > 85% cacao
- ☐ Yogurt
- ☐ Cheese
- ☐ Milk

Avoid these food items on your no sugar journey:

- ☐ Refined flours
- ☐ Condiments
- ☐ Bananas
- ☐ Potatoes

- ☐ Dried fruits, including dates and raisins
- ☐ Artificial sweeteners
- ☐ Beverages like alcohol, soda, sweetened tea, and juices

The Fastest & Easiest Way To Detox & Eliminate Sugar In Only 10 Days To Lose Weight And Burn Fat

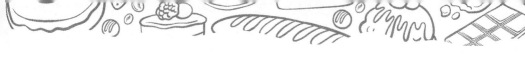

Important Things to Keep in Mind

- **Meat Substitutes**

  Many of you might not want to or cannot eat meat. Nuts and seeds are great healthy protein alternatives to this. Although if you can, I recommend purchasing and eating meat—either organic, grass-fed, or free range with no hormones or antibiotics.

- **Preparing Nuts & Seeds**

  When consuming in large amounts, most nuts and seeds should be soaked, strained, and rinsed before eating. This process eliminates the enzyme inhibitors that can stop their proper absorption.

  These enzyme inhibitors are sometimes referred to as "anti-nutrients" because they can interfere with the process of digestion and cause issues like flatulence and bloating, especially when consumed in large amounts. The main anti-nutrients in nuts and seeds can make it hard to digest the proteins, fats and nutrients. These are called phytates, lectins, oxalates, and enzyme inhibitors.

  However, they can be eliminated or minimized by soaking the seed/nut in pure water, usually overnight or for about 8 hours. This soaking time depends on the specific nut or seed you are going to consume.

  Soft, fattier-type nuts like cashews rarely need soaking for too long. After the soaking period, discard the water and rinse again with fresh water. You can also add salt or lemon juice to the soaking water to help neutralize enzyme inhibitors and reduce the phytic acid, oxalic acid, and lectin content.

  Seeds and nuts, like almonds, pistachios, hazelnuts, sunflower and pumpkin seeds get soft after soaking. You can dehydrate them to create a crunchy snack for yourself.

  Yet another step after soaking your seed/nut is to sprout it slightly. This also significantly reduces the toxic inhibitors that may affect the complete absorption of the nutrients. The process involved is the same as alfalfa sprouts. Use a jar with a mesh lid, then rinse and drain daily until a white sprout emerges from the nut or seed. All varieties won't sprout, but you can experiment with almonds, sunflower and pumpkin seeds.

Different ways to consume soaked nuts and seeds:

★ **Dehydrating:** After soaking for about 8 hours, strain the seeds or nuts and dehydrate them in a dehydrator for several hours. This will give a light, crunchy texture to your seeds and nuts similar to the roasted ones. You can also buy from brand suppliers that pre-soak, pre-sprout, and dehydrate their products for enhanced taste and improved digestibility.

★ **Cultured:** You can culture the nuts and seeds with active lactic acid bacteria, such as a probiotic powder, to produce delicious vegan cheese alternatives.

★ **Blending:** You can further process the soaked and strained seeds to make a variety of foods like desserts, burgers, cheesecakes, or add them to your shake recipes.

• **Water**

Water is the most important nutrient for changing your lifestyle. Most people don't nourish their bodies with adequate amounts of water daily.

Our bodies are made up of 75% water, and we cannot survive more than a few days without it. Problem is that the majority of people have the opinion that drinking teas, juices, sodas, or other drinks will adequately hydrate their body, but this is not true. The reality is that caffeinated drinks are actually diuretics, which causes you to urinate more frequently. This means they dehydrate you even more, so never count your tea or coffee cups towards your number of water glasses per day.

Your daily water requirement depends on your size and weight. Various sources recommend you drink half your weight (in pounds) in ounces of water every day. Using this formula, how much water should a person weighing 130 pounds drink?

Let's calculate! First, divide the weight of the person by 2, 130/2= 65 ounces. This means the person should drink 65 ounces of water every day. Since 8 ounce = 1 glass water, divide 65 ounces with 8 and we get around 8 glasses of water.

So, the formula is simple!

Ounces of water to drink in a day = Your weight in pounds/2

Number of glasses of water to drink in a day = Ounces of water/8

Although, if you are working out or exercising, you might have to drink more water per day.

It is best to drink water on an empty stomach, although this makes scheduling

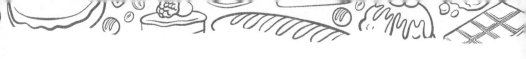

when to drink water a little tricky.

Try this—drink your two glasses of water right when you wake up, drink two more glasses before lunch, then drink two more glasses when you desire your afternoon snack, then drink your last two glasses of water right before dinner. You will go to the bathroom more often if you are not used to drinking this much water. But this is the process of your body expelling toxins.

If you don't consume adequate amounts of water daily, your body will suffer the consequences. Common symptoms of dehydration include fatigue, constipation, dry mouth and skin, kidney and bladder problems, and high blood pressure.

Chapter Summary

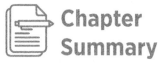

✓ After cleaning out your pantry and refrigerator of all unhealthy food, replace them with healthy food items.

✓ The foods you can actually eat on your no sugar journey are:

- All types of meat and seafood without added sauces or marinade
- All vegetables
- Low-glycemic fruits, like apples, limes, strawberries, apricots, grapefruit, lemon, cantaloupe, guava, nectarines, oranges, pear, watermelon, blueberries, peaches, plums, apples, kiwi, etc.
- All nuts and seeds in raw form
- Legumes and beans
- Whole grains like oats, barley, quinoa, etc.

- All spices
- Sugar-free tea
- Unsweetened almond or nut milk
- Water
- Condiments, such as homemade hot sauce, coconut aminos, apple cider vinegar, red wine vinegar
- Avocado, coconut, and olive oils
- Butter & eggs
- Sugar-free protein powders.

✓ Limit the consumption of monk fruit, stevia, high-glycemic fruits (like cherries, mangoes, prunes, and pineapples), dark chocolate, yogurt, cheese, and milk.

✓ When consuming nuts and seeds in large amounts, make sure to soak them overnight, strain, and rinse before eating. This removes/decreases the enzymatic inhibitors in nuts and seeds.

Drink water in quantities equal to half your weight in ounces every day. It is best to consume water on an empty stomach.

On this journey of going through the sugar detox, you'll be eating differently from how you have normally been eating. The following healthy eating guidelines are some of my secrets to maintaining optimal weight and health.

These guidelines are for a no-sugar eating plan. Such a diet is recommended to prevent and reverse type 2 diabetes, and to improve memory and cognition. This diet also does not raise your blood sugar and insulin levels.

Foods high in carbs causes the release of glucose, which raises your insulin levels, so it is essential to avoid the following: cake, crackers, cookies, sugary cereal and drinks, flour, bread products, jams/jellies, and processed potato products.

Healthy eating guidelines include:

- 50% of your food should come from fresh organic vegetables.

- Eat one fresh serving of any low glycemic fruit per day; only the raw fruit.

- Don't always eat cooked foods. Eat a couple of servings of any raw vegetables every day.

  - If you are eating out, order a salad or raw vegetables for sides.

- 25% of your daily food intake should come from animal or vegetable protein sources. Try to eat fish at least once a week.

- Eat a variety of different nuts and seeds because they are full of minerals, proteins, and essential fatty acids.

- Avoid sugar, flour, rice, pasta and bread. Replace these items with whole grains such as quinoa, amaranth, barley, wild rice, and organic oats.

- Cultured foods such as kimchi, sauerkraut, and plain Greek Yogurt contain probiotics. Adding one to two tablespoons of these foods to your meals is excellent for your health.

- Replace sugary snacks with nuts, seeds, nut butter (excluding peanut butter), and berries.

- Replace condiments and sauces containing MSG or high fructose corn syrup with vinegar, spices, and herbs.

- Replace table salt with kosher, sea salt, or pink Himalayan salt.
- Replace fried foods with baked foods.
- Remember to chew your food thoroughly so your saliva coats all of the food you are eating in order to aid in your digestion.

How to ease withdrawal symptoms when you quit sugar?

Going on this sugar detox can lower your risk for diabetes, help you lose weight, and clear up and brighten your skin.

However, quitting sugar is not easy for most people, especially at first. I have never had a single client who didn't have any trouble cutting out sugar. As discussed in the first chapter on how powerful and addictive sugar can be, this is not too surprising.

It follows, then, that eliminating sugar from your diet can bring some less than pleasant side effects. For the people who are really dependent, they will feel strong withdrawal symptoms such as crankiness, irritability, fatigue or headaches.

So, how do you keep these symptoms at bay and control your sweet cravings?

- **Cut it out all at once**

The best way to cut out sugar is to go cold turkey. Telling a severe sugar addict to slowly reduce the amount of sugar each day is like telling an alcoholic to drink less.

Cutting out sugar all at once lowers the risk that you will bend the rules by opting to eat a cookie over here or a doughnut over there. Initially, you have to eliminate sugar completely from your diet for a full three days, even the sugar found in dairy and fruits.

The first three days will be rough, but this is the minimum time needed to break old habits and establish the new ones. After three days, you can slowly start incorporating fruits in your diet.

- **Eat good to feel good**

Once your usual supply of sugar gets cut, your body will probably rebel by messing with your mood and energy levels.

I stress to my clients the importance of nourishing yourself with high quality foods that can help fight moodiness and energize you when you cut out the sweets.

Keep yourself satisfied with foods high in fat such as fish, nuts, and avocados. I also recommend and remind my clients to drink plenty of water. This can help fight fatigue and headaches, which are other side effects of going cold turkey on sugar.

Eating lots of vegetables and organic protein will keep you feeling full and keep your appetite under control. To avoid feeling hungry throughout the day, munch on snacks that deliver good fats and fiber such as celery and guacamole or carrots and hummus.

- **Combat your cravings the right way**

Since you will fight off a host of emotional and physical side effects on this diet, your body will play mean tricks on you by kicking your sugar cravings hard.

If you are craving for a hot fudge sundae, try spicing up your savory food instead. Just because you are going sugar free does not mean your food has to taste bland. Use lots of herbs and spices and ingredients such as garlic, onion, and lime to help you cut out your sugar without feeling like your food tastes terrible.

Another strategy is to have unsweetened iced tea or cold brew. Cold drinks really help curb sugar cravings.

- **Add natural sugar back slowly**

After your first three days on the sugar detox, it's okay to incorporate foods that contain natural sugar like fruits. But when you take your first bite, expect it to taste a little different and sweeter. After three days, your palate has basically been recalibrated.

Eating sugary foods actually diminishes the ability to taste sweetness, so avoiding sugar for three days will actually make naturally sweet foods more satisfying and sweet.

However, I recommend adding natural sugars back slowly, such as one or two servings of fruit per day. Adding them back slowly to your diet will ease the withdrawal symptoms by not making you crave added sugars that you gave up only a couple of days ago. Soon, your body will adjust to lower levels of only natural sugar and you will successfully have detoxed!

The best news is that you don't have to give up your fudge sundae forever. At the

The Fastest & Easiest Way To Detox & Eliminate Sugar
In Only 10 Days To Lose Weight And Burn Fat

end of every week, you can have an intentional indulgence. It can be a cupcake or a snack of French fries. I have found that completely depriving yourself of an entire food group can end poorly. If we fully restrict ourselves long-term, we can set up ourselves for failure and make bad decisions, such as not sticking to the diet after about a month.

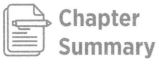

Chapter Summary

✓ The no-sugar diet plan is recommended to prevent and reverse type 2 diabetes, improve your memory and cognition, and help you lose weight.

✓ While on this sugar detox journey, you are required to follow the healthy eating guidelines given in the chapter.

✓ Always chew your food thoroughly so that your saliva coats the food you eat and to help with proper digestion.

✓ Since sugar is addictive, quitting sugar for the first time is not easy for most people. They experience strong withdrawal symptoms like crankiness, fatigue, irritability, and headaches.

✓ To ease these withdrawal symptoms, cut out all sugar from your diet at once, even the natural sugars from dairy and fruits for full three days.

• After three days, incorporate sugars from natural sources like fruits slowly.

✓ Eat fresh vegetables and protein-rich foods throughout your detox journey to feel good, ease your withdrawal symptoms, and keep sugar cravings at bay. Also, drink the required amount of water per day.

08 Starting The Sugar Detox: Day 1-3

As we said earlier, you'll begin your sugar detox journey by cutting out all sugar for the first three days, even from fruits. These three days help reset your sugar cravings. After these three days, you can add fruits back to your diet slowly.

However, the first three days are the hardest because most recipes have sugar or fruits in them. Therefore, I have gathered some best recipes that taste amazing and are fairly easy to cook.

Although I have listed the recipes according to the days, you can mix and match these fresh meals. For example, if you want to eat Day 2's dinner on Day 1, you can make it for dinner on Day 1. But if the meal is labeled a snack, then only eat that one snack for the day. Don't eat snacks on Day 1 for breakfast, then snacks on Day 2 for lunch.

On the sugar detox, you do not have to limit the amount of food you eat. Since these recipes are fresh and healthy, you need not worry about the calories as well. Remember, this detox is all about cutting sugar. If you are hungry, eat your meal until you are full.

We are not trying to restrict how much you eat. We're just cutting out the sugars, and giving your body the right food it needs to be healthy. So, eat as much of these healthy foods until you are completely satisfied and full!

DAY 01

Breakfast:
Overnight Oats

Ingredients:

- 1/2 cup oats
- 1/2 cup almond milk
- 1 tsp. crushed almond
- 1 tsp. hemp seeds
- 1/4 tsp. cinnamon

Directions:

1. Place oats into a small bowl or jar.
2. Pour almond milk over the oats.
3. Add the other ingredients and leave in the refrigerator overnight to enjoy it for breakfast.

Snack:
Quick Black Bean Hummus With Vegetables

Black beans are a delicious and healthy alternative to the usual garbanzo beans in hummus. This recipe is a nice staple for any occasion or family gathering. If you have any roasted veggies on hand, they can make a significant addition blended into the hummus.

Ingredients:

- 2 (15 ounce) cans black beans, drained
- 6 cloves garlic, minced
- 1 teaspoon tahini
- 2 teaspoons lemon juice
- 1 teaspoon ground cumin
- 1 pinch salt and ground black pepper to taste
- 2 tablespoons olive oil, or to taste

Directions:

1. Blend the black beans, garlic, lemon juice, tahini, cumin, salt, and black pepper together in a blender.
2. Pour olive oil into the blender in a steady stream until it reaches the desired consistency.

🔅 **Tips** ───────────────────────────────

✓ You can substitute crushed garlic with fresh garlic, if desired.

✓ You can reserve and use some bean liquid mixed with the olive oil to cut down on fat content.

✓ You can store this snack in the refrigerator for 2 to 3 weeks

 Lunch:
Refreshing Red Cabbage Salad

Red cabbage is great for your gut health. The insoluble fiber in red cabbage promotes regularity and relieves symptoms of any gastrointestinal disorders.

The red hue that makes red cabbage so vibrant actually comes from a plant-based chemical called flavonoids. It not only provides the cabbage with a beautiful color, but it is also the source of fiber, essential vitamins, and minerals.

1 cup of red cabbage has 56% of the daily recommended intake of Vitamin C.

Ingredients:

Salad:

- 2 cups red cabbage (thinly sliced)
- 2 cups shredded carrots
- 2 cups shredded cucumber (deseeded)
- 1 cup parsley
- 1/4 cup or 2 tablespoons roasted, unsalted pumpkin seeds
- 1/4 cup or 2 Tablespoons unsalted sunflower seeds

Lemon Tahini Parsley Dressing:

- Juice of 1 1/2 lemons
- 3 tablespoons apple cider vinegar
- 4 tablespoons tahini
- 3 tablespoons coconut nectar
- 1/4 cup avocado oil
- 1 small garlic clove
- 1/4 cup fresh parsley
- Salt and pepper to taste

Directions:

1. Slice the red cabbage very thin lengthwise and cut these thin slices again into half.
2. Shred the peeled carrots and deseeded cucumber and finely chop the parsley.
3. Mix the red cabbage, carrots, cucumber, parsley, and pumpkin and sunflower seeds in a bowl.
4. To make the dressing for the cabbage salad, place all the dressing ingredients into your food processor and blend until smooth. Add more coconut nectar, tahini, or avocado oil according to your taste.
5. Once the dressing is ready, mix all of it into the cabbage salad bowl, and garnish with fresh parsley leaves. Enjoy your salad immediately.

Dinner:
Sheet Pan Chicken and Asparagus Bowl

Using only 4 main ingredients and 25 minutes to cook, I absolutely love this recipe for its simplicity. Simple doesn't mean bland because the chicken in this recipe is seasoned with savory oyster sauce and minced fresh garlic!

Ingredients:

- Oil spray
- 1.5 lbs chicken, boneless, skinless thigh or breast
- 1 lb asparagus with tough ends trimmed

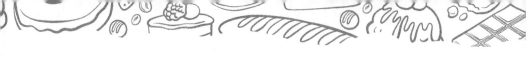

- 1/4 cup oyster sauce
- 2 cloves garlic, minced

Directions:

1. Preheat the oven to 425° F. Line a baking sheet with aluminum foil for an easy clean. Spray on a thin layer of oil.
2. Arrange asparagus onto the baking sheet without overlapping. Place chicken on the stem side of the asparagus without overlapping.
3. Mix oyster sauce and minced garlic in a small bowl. Brush over the chicken and the asparagus.
4. Bake until the chicken is cooked through, about 20 minutes.
5. Serve hot.

DAY 02

Breakfast:
Mixed Grain Cereal with Chai Spice
Servings: Serves 4

Ingredients:

Cereal:

- 1 cup combination of whole grains, like millet, barley, spelt, kamut, flaxseed, and steel-cut oats
- 1 tbsp. grated fresh ginger
- 1 cinnamon stick
- Seeds from 6 cardamom pods or 1/2 tsp. ground cardamom
- 1/4 tsp. coarsely ground black pepper
- 1/4 tsp. sea salt

For serving:

- Almond milk
- Chopped almonds

Directions:

You can prepare the recipe in advance and heat a portion in the morning for breakfast. It will keep in the refrigerator for a week.

1. In a medium saucepan, boil 3 cups of water. Turn off the heat once boiled.
2. Add grains, ginger, cinnamon, cardamom, pepper, and salt. Cover and let

it stand 2 hours or overnight.

3. In the morning, set the pan over medium heat, bring to a boil, reduce to low, and simmer until the grains are tender; about 15 minutes (this will vary depending on the soak time)

4. Discard the cinnamon stick. Divide the cereal among 4 bowls, and serve with warm almond milk and chopped almonds.

Snack:
Guacamole with vegetables

Ingredients:

- 3 avocados - peeled, pitted, and mashed
- Juice of 1 lemon
- 1 teaspoon salt
- 1/2 cup diced onion
- 3 tablespoons chopped fresh cilantro
- 2 roma (plum) tomatoes, diced
- 1 teaspoon minced garlic
- 1 pinch ground cayenne pepper (optional)

Directions:

1. In a medium bowl, mix the avocados, lime juice, and salt.
2. Mix in onion, cilantro, tomatoes, and garlic.
3. Stir in cayenne pepper.
4. Refrigerate for 1 hour for best flavor, or serve immediately.

Lunch:
Blackened Chicken and Avocado Salad

Ingredients:

The blackened chicken:

- 2 boneless, skinless chicken breasts, sliced horizontally
- 1/2 teaspoon paprika
- 1/2 teaspoon garlic powder
- 1/2 teaspoon chili powder
- 1/2 teaspoon cumin, optional
- 1/2 teaspoon powdered chicken stock, optional
- 1 tablespoon olive oil
- Pinch of salt and fresh cracked pepper (coarsely ground black pepper)

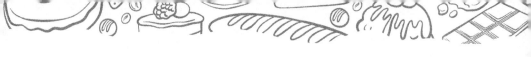

The avocado salad:

- 2 cups chopped romaine lettuce
- 1 cup cherry tomatoes, halved
- 1 small onion, chopped
- 2 avocados
- 1 tablespoon olive oil
- 1 tablespoon chopped cilantro, fresh or dried
- Salt and fresh cracked pepper, to taste
- Parmesan shavings, optional

Directions:

1. In a small bowl, mix the paprika, garlic powder, chili powder, cumin, salt, pepper, and olive oil. Coat the chicken breasts with the marinade and cook on medium-low heat in a skillet until cooked through. If chicken browns too fast, reduce the heat.

2. Add the chopped lettuce, diced avocado, tomato, and onion to a large salad bowl, drizzling the olive oil and sprinkling with salt, pepper, and cilantro. Toss to combine and sprinkle with parmesan shavings. You can also add a good drizzle of apple cider vinegar dressing.

3. Once cooked, transfer cooked chicken breasts to a cutting board and cut into ½-inch strips, place on top of the avocado salad, and serve immediately.

 Tips For The Blackened Chicken Salad

Blackening spices change this protein-rich salad into a flavor explosion in every bite without adding tons of fat or calories. Here are a few tips on how to make this blackened chicken salad:

✓ Slice the chicken breasts horizontally so they cook faster. You can also use chicken tenders.

✓ Chopped cucumber, crispy bacon, and olives make for a great addition to this salad.

✓ To keep avocados from turning brown, brush them with lemon juice. It will act as an antioxidant and keep the avocados from turning brown too quickly.

✓ Being a cold chicken salad, this recipe is perfect for summers, picnics, or potlucks. You can make it up a day in advance, leaving the avocado and tomato until you are ready to serve the chicken salad.

Dinner:
Sheet Pan Chicken Fajita Bowl

Ingredients:

- 1.5 lbs chicken breasts, boneless, skinless
- Olive oil to taste
- 1 tbsp taco seasoning
- 3 ea bell peppers sliced
- 1 ea onion, sliced thinly
- Fresh limes

Directions:

1. Preheat the oven to 400° F and grease a large rimmed baking sheet.
2. Slice the chicken into strips and season to coat with taco seasoning. Lightly drizzle the seasoned chicken with olive oil.
3. Chop all veggies into strips. Drizzle with olive oil and more taco seasoning if required.
4. Place the chicken and veggies on the sheet pan and bake at 400° F until chicken strips are cooked through and veggies are tender, about 20-25 minutes.
5. Remove from the oven and squeeze fresh lime over. Serve as desired in tortillas or over cauliflower rice.

DAY 03

Breakfast:
Tomato Grits and Sausage Recipe

Serves 6

Ingredients:

- 3 cups low-sodium chicken broth
- 1 can (10 ounces) Ro-Tel or other diced tomatoes with chiles
- 1 cup quick-cooking grits
- 3/4 cup grated low-fat Cheddar cheese
- 8 ounces turkey kielbasa, coarsely chopped
- 1/2 cup coarsely chopped scallions (white and light green parts only), for serving

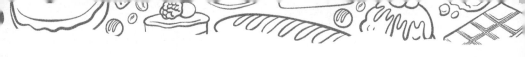

Directions:

1. In a medium saucepan, bring the chicken broth and tomatoes to a boil over medium-high heat. Slowly whisk in the grits, reduce the heat to low, and cook, stirring until thickened, 6 to 8 minutes. Add in the Cheddar cheese and remove from the heat.

2. Meanwhile, in a medium nonstick skillet, cook the sausage over medium heat, stirring until browned all over, 5 to 7 minutes. Stir half of the sausage into the grits.

3. Spoon the grits into bowls and top with the remaining sausage and the scallions.

Snack:
Granola + Plain Greek Yogurt

Ingredients:

- 3 3/4 cups rolled oats
- 1/2 cup chopped almonds
- 1/4 cup dried, unsweetened coconut
- 1/4 cup sesame seeds
- 2 teaspoons ground cinnamon
- 1/4 teaspoon salt
- 3 large egg whites
- 1 teaspoon vanilla extract

Directions:

1. Preheat the oven to 225° F (110° C). Line a baking sheet with parchment paper.

2. Combine oats, almonds, coconut, sesame seeds, cinnamon, and salt in a large bowl.

3. Beat egg whites in a bowl until stiff peaks form. Add vanilla extract. Fold egg whites into the oat mixture. Spread on the prepared baking sheet.

4. Bake in the preheated oven, stirring every 20 minutes until granola is crispy; about 1 hour.

Lunch:
Carrot Meatballs with Mint Cauliflower Rice

Ingredients:

For the Meatballs:

- 1 lb. lean ground beef, chicken or turkey
- 1 large egg
- 1/2 cup grated carrots
- 1 tsp. Italian seasoning
- 1/2 tsp. crushed red pepper flakes
- Salt & pepper to taste
- 2 tbsp. extra-virgin olive oil

For the Cauliflower Rice:

- 4 cups riced cauliflower
- 1 tbsp. lemon juice
- 4 mint leaves
- Salt & pepper to taste
- 1/2 cup water

Directions:

1. In a large bowl, whisk egg with Italian seasoning, salt, pepper, and red pepper flakes.
2. Add carrots and ground meat to the bowl. Using your hands, mix the ingredients thoroughly throughout the meat. Using a small ice-cream scoop, roll the meat into balls.
3. Heat a medium skillet over medium-high heat. Add oil to the pan and heat for 4 minutes, then add the meatballs to the pan.
4. Cook meatballs for 5 minutes, then flip to cook on the other side for 5 minutes. Rotate the meatballs a few more times in the pan, cooking 1-2 minutes until cooked through. Remove meatballs from the pan and place on a plate.
5. Add 1/4 cup water to the skillet with riced cauliflower. Cook for 5 minutes until softened, then add lemon juice and mint leaves. Stir to combine.
6. Divide the meatballs and cauliflower rice into 4 even servings placing them in meal prep containers with fresh lemon wedges.

Dinner:
15 Minute Sesame Salmon with Bok Choy and Mushrooms

Ingredients:

Main Dish:

- 4 each 4-6 oz. salmon fillet
- 2 each portobello mushroom caps (or 8 oz. baby bella mushrooms)
- 4 each baby bok choy
- 1 tbsp toasted sesame seeds
- 1 each green onion

For the Cauliflower Rice:

- 1 tbsp olive oil
- 1 tsp sesame oil
- 1 tbsp Coconut Amino
- 1/2-inch Ginger, grated (approx. 1 tsp.)
- 1/2 lemon juice
- 1/2 tsp salt
- 1/2 tsp black pepper

Directions:

1. Whisk together all the marinade ingredients.
2. Drizzle half of the marinade on the salmon and turn to coat. Cover and refrigerate the salmon while it marinates for one hour.
3. Preheat the oven to 400° F.
4. Prepare the vegetables: Trim the rough ends from the bok choy and cut into halves. Slice the mushrooms into ½ inch pieces.
5. Drizzle the remaining marinade over the vegetables and lay on a lined baking sheet.
6. Place salmon, skin side down, on a lined baking sheet as well. Bake until salmon is cooked through, about 20 minutes.
7. Top with sliced green onions and sesame seeds.

Along with these recipes, remember to have your daily water intake as well for each day. This is very important.

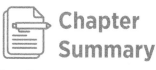

Chapter Summary

✓ The first three days of sugar detox are the hardest and leave you wondering what to eat if you have to cut out all sugar in your diet.

- However, going on a sugar detox doesn't mean you have to stop eating or reduce your meal intake.

✓ Substitute your meals and snacks with healthy, sugar-free recipes given in the chapter for the first three days.

✓ Remember, not to ditch water and drink adequate amounts daily to keep with your recommended intake.

Nightmare Withdrawals: Days 4-7

Congratulations on getting through the first 3 days successfully! I know these first 3 days were the hardest because you had absolutely no sugar.

Now, your cravings and withdrawal symptoms might have started to pop up. Therefore, I have provided you with recipes with small amounts of fruit to be eaten daily! At this point of time, it is important for you to have little amounts of fruit to satisfy your sugar cravings and not make you want to stop your diet entirely.

It's important to continue eating healthy after the first three days of the sugar detox by incorporating sugar from natural sources like fruits, but do so slowly. However, eating fruits does need not be boring with your recipes.

DAY 04

Breakfast:
Oatmeal Pancake with Berries

Ingredients:

- 1/2 cup rolled oats
- 3 or 4 egg whites
- 1/4 of an apple, grated
- Cinnamon, to taste
- Fresh berries, for serving
- Cooking spray

Directions:

1. Mix all the ingredients together in a medium bowl to form a medium consistency batter. Leave it for 5 to 10 minutes.

2. Heat a nonstick pan over medium heat, and coat with the cooking spray. Ladle spoonfuls of batter onto the pan. Cook on a medium heat till both the sides are golden brown.

3. Serve with fresh berries.

Snack:

Avocado Banana Smoothie

It's a creamy avocado smoothie that's easy to prepare, requiring just **5 ingredients, 1 blender, and 5 minutes.**

Frozen banana creates a creamy and naturally sweet base for the smoothie. Avocados are full of fiber and healthy fats, which makes this smoothie almost like a milkshake.

I recommend using dairy-free milk for the recipe. Protein powder is the final ingredient which makes this smoothie a proper meal.

Ingredients:

- 1 large frozen banana (ripe, peeled, and sliced)
- 1/4 – 1/2 medium ripe avocado
- 1 scoop plain or vanilla protein powder
- 1 large handful greens of choice (spinach, kale, rainbow chard)
- 3/4 – 1 cup unsweetened plain almond milk or any dairy-free milk
- 1 tbsp seed of choice (hemp, flax, sesame, sunflower, chia, etc.) (optional)
- 1/2 tsp ashwagandha (optional)
- 1/2 cup sliced frozen (or fresh) cucumber or berries (organic when possible)

Directions:

1. Add frozen banana, avocado, protein powder, greens, and dairy-free milk to a blender. Further add the seeds, ashwagandha or additional fruits and vegetables (such as berries or cucumbers).

2. Blend on high until creamy and smooth, scraping down the sides occasionally. If smoothie is too thick, add more dairy-free milk to it. If too thin, add more frozen banana or avocado.

3. Taste and adjust the flavor as needed, adding more banana for sweetness, avocado for creaminess, or greens for vibrant green color. Protein powder can also be used to add more sweetness.

4. Enjoy your smoothie fresh. Leftovers can be kept covered in the refrigerator up to 24 hours or in the freezer up to 2 weeks.

Lunch:
Skillet Shrimp with Tomato & Avocado

Shrimps are a low-calorie, low-fat source of protein.

Ingredients:

- 2 tbsp ghee or grass-fed butter
- 1 lbs Shrimp, peeled
- 1/2 tsp dried parsley
- Salt and pepper to taste
- 4 ea Scallions, chopped and separated into white and green sections
- 1 lbs tomatoes, seeded and diced
- 3 cloves garlic, minced
- 1-2 tsp chipotle peppers in adobo sauce, minced
- 1 ea Avocado, seeded and diced
- 1 tbsp lime juice
- 1/4 cup Fresh cilantro, chopped

Directions:

1. Heat the ghee or butter in a skillet over medium-high heat.
2. Season the shrimp with 1/2 teaspoon of dried parsley, salt, and pepper. Place the shrimp in the hot pan and cook for a minute. Flip the shrimp over and cook again.
3. Next, add tomatoes, white scallion parts, minced garlic, and minced chipotle. Cook everything for a minute or two until shrimp turns opaque.
4. Remove from heat and add in the diced avocados, green scallion parts, lime juice, and cilantro. Serve immediately.

Dinner:
Spicy Mustard Thyme Chicken & Coconut Roasted Brussel Sprouts

Ingredients:

- 1 lb. Brussel sprouts, sliced in half
- 2 medium boneless, skinless chicken breasts
- 1/4 cup ground spicy mustard
- 1 tbsp. lemon juice
- 1 tsp. thyme
- Salt & pepper to taste
- 1 tbsp. melted coconut oil

Directions:

1. In a small bowl, whisk the spicy mustard with lemon juice, salt, pepper and thyme.

2. Place the two chicken breasts in a bowl and pour the mustard over them. Coat the chicken breasts with the mustard using a spoon. Keep this in the refrigerator to marinate for 10 minutes. Then remove and bring to room temperature 15 minutes prior to cooking.

3. Preheat the oven to 350° F. Prepare a baking sheet with parchment paper.

4. Place the Brussel sprouts in a medium bowl and toss with melted coconut oil, salt, and pepper.

5. Transfer the sprouts to the prepared baking sheets, spreading into an even layer.

6. Place the marinated chicken breasts in a glass baking pan and bake for 10 minutes.

7. After 10 minutes, place the Brussel sprouts in the oven. Cook both for 15 minutes.

8. Remove from the oven and serve the meal hot.

DAY 05

Breakfast:
Strawberry Coconut Yogurt

Ingredients:

Coconut Yogurt:

- 1 cup of Greek Yogurt
- 1 tbsp of Coconut Milk

Toppings:

- 5 Sliced Strawberries
- 1 tbsp. of Chia Seeds
- 1 tbsp. of Unsweetened, Shredded Coconut
- 1/2 tbsp. of Hemp Seeds
- 1/2 tbsp. of Sunflower Seeds
- 1 tbsp. of natural Peanut Butter

Directions:

1. Mix yogurt, coconut milk, and maple syrup in a medium bowl
2. Top with sliced strawberries, chia, coconut, hemp seeds, sunflower seeds and peanut butter.
3. Enjoy your breakfast.

Snack:
Watermelon Slushy

Every function in our body—from digestion to brain function and respiratory health—rely on sufficient water intake to work properly. However, drinking plain water every day is not enticing for many, so I've come up with this simple, refreshing watermelon slushy to keep you hydrated!

Importance of staying hydrated

1. For Skin

Like any other organ of your body, your skin is made up of cells which require water to function optimally. Dehydration can result in skin problems, from acne to wrinkles.

Plus, water is essential for the release of toxins, particularly through our digestive system. So, keeping your water intake high will help prevent skin breakouts.

2. For your Heart

Water also eases your blood flow through the arteries and veins, thus improving circulation. This ensures that your heart is not working in overdrive to move your blood throughout your body and encourages blood flow to your skin, giving you a healthy glow.

3. For Healthy Weight

You feel thirsty when your body is dehydrated. Loss of even 2-3 % of water slows down your organ functions and decreases your metabolism. Kidneys are the first organ to slow down when you are dehydrated, pushing the workload on the liver. The liver is responsible for the breakdown of fat in your body; and when it is overwhelmed by the decrease in kidney functions, your fat-burning mechanism gets affected.

4. For your Brain

Your brain vitally relies on water to function optimally (our brains are made up of about eighty percent water). When there's water loss in the body, your cognitive function decreases, which results in a feeling of low energy or even exhaustion. This makes you move less and crave food, particularly simple carbohydrates and sugar, which our body views as quick energy sources.

With chronic dehydration, you tend to lose energy, which can result in weight gain over time. This can be a 4-6-pound weight gain over a year just from not consuming enough water.

Hydration Also Comes from Food

During hotter months, water-dense produce comes into season. Juicy fruits like pineapple, mango, greens, and watermelon are the major produce of the summer season. Watermelon contains over ninety-two percent water, which is why this recipe doesn't call for any liquid. It also contains many micronutrients like potassium (more than a banana), which is a crucial mineral for regulating fluids in the body.

Serves 2

Ingredients:

- 1/2 watermelon (2-2.5 lbs)
- 1/4 cup fresh mint
- 1 lime, juiced
- 2 cups ice
- Optional: 1-2 tablespoons chia seeds

Directions:

1. Cut watermelon in half and scoop out from one side. Remove stems from mint leaves and discard. Cut lime in half and juice both sides.

2. Add all ingredients to the blender and blend until smooth.

3. Serve immediately!

Lunch:
Summer Salad

We all want fresh and light produce in summers. And what better way to satisfy that craving than a colorful, nutritious salad? This recipe uses the best of the season's flavors—spicy radishes, cleansing greens, juicy nectarines, and crunchy snap peas. You can also add a protein of your choice to this dish. This summer salad makes you feel satisfied without feeling weighed down.

Recipe Ingredients:

- **Arugula**

  Arugula is packed with nutrients, especially high amounts of folic acid, which is particularly beneficial for pregnant women. It has been shown to prevent certain birth defects and keep blood pressure down during pregnancy. Moreover, it plays a significant role in red cell production in the human body. Folic acid helps prevent anemia and chronic illnesses like cancer. In addition to its nutrient density, it gives a spicy flavor to your salad.

- **Snap Peas**

  Snap peas add the fresh, crispy texture the summer salad calls for. Being rich in Vitamin K, they are crucial for bone and heart health, blood clotting, and brain health. They are also an excellent plant source of iron, which is important for creating new cells and preventing anemia. Iron deficiency can lead to chronic fatigue, hair loss, muscle weakness, and poor circulation. The beta-carotene found in snap peas
  and prevents cancer.

- **Salad Dressing**

  This summer salad is rich in fat-soluble vitamins A, D, E, and K. Fat-soluble vitamins require adequate fat consumption to be fully utilized by the body. The olive oil in the dressing provides healthy fats to keep you satiated, and helps your body utilize the nutrients from the produce. The dressing also contains mustard which helps prevent cancer, improves skin health, and can even help with muscle pain.

Ingredients:

Dressing:

- 2 teaspoons Dijon mustard
- 1 tablespoon finely minced shallots
- 1/4 cup white wine vinegar or champagne vinegar
- 1/2 teaspoon kosher salt
- 1/4 cup extra-virgin olive oil
- Fresh ground black pepper to taste

Salad:

- 5 ounces arugula and spinach mix (or just arugula)
- 4 ounces snap peas
- 2 nectarines
- 1/2 cup radishes
- 1/4 cup pine nuts
- 1/4 cup mint

Directions:

1. Take one teaspoon of olive oil in a sauté pan over medium-low heat. Add the pine nuts and toast, constantly tossing until light brown (don't step away from the pan as they burn easily).

2. To make the dressing, finely mince the shallots and shake or whisk with the other dressing ingredients.

3. Wash and dry the arugula mix. Thinly slice the radishes. Wash the snap peas. Thinly slice the nectarines. Pick mint leaves from the stem and chop.

4. Add all the ingredients to a large serving bowl.

5. When you're ready to serve, toss with the dressing (add only ¼ of the dressing at a time to prevent overdressing). Store remaining dressing in the refrigerator. Enjoy!

Dinner:
Roast Pork with Apples & Onions

Ingredients:

- 1 boneless pork loin roast (2 pounds)
- 1/4 teaspoon salt
- 1/4 teaspoon pepper
- 1 tablespoon olive oil
- 3 large golden delicious apples, cut into 1-inch wedges
- 2 large onions, cut into 3/4-inch wedges
- 5 garlic cloves, peeled
- 1 tablespoon minced fresh rosemary or 1 teaspoon dried rosemary, crushed

Directions:

1. Preheat the oven to 350° F. Sprinkle pork loin roast with salt and pepper.

2. In a large nonstick skillet, heat oil over medium heat, brown roast pork loin on all sides.

3. Transfer to a roasting pan coated with cooking spray. Place apples, onions and garlic around the roast; sprinkle with rosemary.

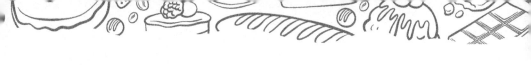

Breakfast:
Mango Coconut Chia Pudding (Make this the night before!)

Benefits of Chia Seeds

Chia seeds are rich in Omega fatty acids which help to decrease inflammation in the body, promote cell regeneration, and help with brain function. Fiber in the seeds keeps your digestive system functioning optimally, which prevents constipation.

Ingredients:

- 2 cups canned coconut milk
- 1/2 cup chia seeds
- 2 cups chopped mango (frozen is fine)

Directions:

1. Add all ingredients into a sealed container and shake. Keep it in the refrigerator overnight (or at least 6 hours).
2. Garnish with cinnamon (optional) and serve immediately.

Snack:
Kale Chips

Kale is denser than other green leafy vegetables, making it hard for some to digest in its raw form. Sautéing is the most common form of cooking kale, but you can also turn it into crispy, flavorful chips.

Kale's texture makes it perfect for creating crunchy chips that don't fall apart.

Kale belongs to the Brassica family, along with Brussels sprouts and cabbage, and is dense in many nutrients. Its role in our detoxification system is one of the greatest benefits of consuming kale on a regular basis.

Kale further improves your cardiovascular health. Specifically, kale can decrease cholesterol levels. The fiber in kale binds with the bile acids found in the digestive tract, making it easier for bile to be excreted and do its job of breaking down fats.

Kale is also one of the densest sources of lutein, an antioxidant commonly known for its benefits for our eye health. We can't create this antioxidant on our own, so it's important to consume it through food. Lutein has been shown to stop or slow the progression of certain eye diseases. This antioxidant also helps in preventing skin diseases and certain cancers.

Ingredients:

- 1 large bunch curly kale
- 2 teaspoons olive oil
- 1 heaping tablespoon nutritional yeast
- 1 teaspoon garlic powder
- 1/2 teaspoon paprika
- 1/8-1/4 teaspoon salt
- Cayenne pepper, to taste

Directions:

1. Heat the oven to 300° F. Wash and dry kale. Remember to dry every bit of water off the kale. If you leave them moist, the kale will steam in the oven and the chips will turn out soggy.

2. Massage every nook and cranny of the kale with olive oil, one teaspoon at a time. It's important not to drown the kale in oil and to distribute the oil evenly.

3. Mix all the spices together and sprinkle over kale. Toss until fully combined.

4. Spread kale onto a parchment paper-lined baking sheet. Bake for 20-25 minutes, tossing half-way through. When you take the chips out of the oven, they may still feel slightly soft. Let them cool for 10 minutes and they'll turn crispy.

Lunch:
Garlic Butter Chicken Meatballs with Cauliflower Rice

Ingredients:

- 1 lb (450g) ground chicken (or turkey)
- 1/2 cup shredded cheese of your choice (mozzarella, cheddar, provolone...)
- 4 cloves garlic, grated + 2 cloves garlic, minced
- 1 teaspoon Italian seasoning
- 1/2 teaspoon red crushed chili pepper flakes, optional
- 1 crumbled bouillon cube, optional
- 1/2 cup chicken stock
- Salt and fresh cracked black pepper, to taste
- 1/2 cup freshly chopped parsley (or cilantro)
- 3 tablespoons butter, divided

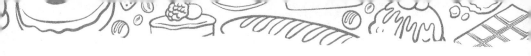

- Juice of 1/2 lemon
- 1 tablespoon hot sauce of your choice
- 1 medium cauliflower head, grated

Directions:

1. Make cauliflower rice with a large grater or food processor. Transfer to a shallow plate with 1/2 cup water and cook covered in the microwave for 4 minutes.

2. In a large bowl, combine ground chicken, cheese, grated garlic, Italian seasoning, crumbled bouillon cube, red chili pepper flakes, chopped cilantro, and black pepper. Mix well and form medium balls. Arrange on a plate and set aside.

3. Melt 2 tablespoons butter in a large skillet over medium-low heat. Cook the chicken meatballs for 8 – 10 minutes on all sides, until brown and cooked through. While cooking, baste the meatballs with the mix of butter and juices. Remove to a clean plate and set aside.

4. In the same skillet, melt the remaining butter. Add lemon juice, chicken stock, hot sauce, minced garlic, parsley, and red pepper flakes (if you want). Cook for 3 or 4 minutes, stirring regularly until the sauce has reduced a bit. Adjust seasoning with salt and pepper, and garnish with more cilantro or parsley if you like.

5. Divide cauliflower rice into meal prep containers. Then top with chicken meatballs and garnish with lemon slices. Drizzle a bit of the sauce over the meatballs and cauliflower rice, or keep the sauce into small containers. Reheat quickly in the microwave when ready to eat.

Dinner:
20-Minute Baked Pesto Salmon

Ingredients:

For the Salmon Packs:

- 9 ounces salmon or 3 filets
- 1 bunch asparagus ~6 cups
- 3 tsp extra-virgin olive oil
- Salt and pepper to taste

For the Pesto:

- 1 avocado, ripe
- 1 parsley, roughly chopped
- 1/2 tsp red pepper flakes
- 2 tbsp extra-virgin olive oil
- 1/2 tsp sea salt
- 1/2 tsp garlic powder

Directions:

1. Preheat the oven to 375° F. Prepare a baking sheet by placing 3 sheets of tin foil on them. The tin foil pieces should be large enough to cover 6-7 asparagus & salmon each.

2. Add all the ingredients for the pesto in a blender except the extra-virgin olive oil. Blend on high until creamy, then slowly drizzle in the extra-virgin olive oil to emulsify.

3. Next, place 6-7 asparagus on one foil, drizzle with 1 tsp of extra-virgin olive oil, sprinkle salt & pepper. Top the asparagus with a salmon fillet. Then, smooth 1 tablespoon of the pesto over the top of the salmon.

4. Close the foil over the salmon and asparagus by bringing the two sides together and crinkling the edges together. Crinkle the top and bottom as well until it is closed completely.

5. Repeat the process for the remaining 2 salmon fillets.

6. Place the foil packets on the baking sheet. Bake for 20 minutes until the salmon is flaky.

7. Serve immediately with extra pesto on the side!

DAY 07

Breakfast:
Healthy 2 Ingredient Pancakes

Ingredients:

- 2 medium ripe banana
- 2 medium eggs
- Butter or oil for the pan

Optional extras:

- 2-3 tablespoons almond meal
- 1 tablespoon cocoa powder or protein powder
- 1/4 teaspoon baking powder for fluffy pancakes
- 1/4 teaspoon vanilla
- 1/4 cup fresh berries
- A pinch of cinnamon

The Fastest & Easiest Way To Detox & Eliminate Sugar
In Only 10 Days To Lose Weight And Burn Fat

Directions:

1. Peel the banana and break up into several big chunks in a bowl. Gently mash the bananas into smaller chunks using a fork.

2. Add the eggs to the mashed bananas and stir with the fork until you have a custard-like consistency. The batter will be runny and should have a few clumps of bananas. *(optional: add 1/4 teaspoon baking powder, 1/4 teaspoon vanilla, pinch of cinnamon, 1 tablespoon cocoa-powder)*

3. Heat a griddle over medium heat and melt about ¼ teaspoon of butter in the pan. Drop about 2 tablespoons of the batter on a hot griddle. Add the nuts, chocolate chips or berries if desired.

4. Cook till the bottoms are golden brown.

5. Gently flip the pancakes and cook for another minute on the other side. Transfer the cooked pancakes to a serving plate and continue cooking the rest of the batter.

6. Serve the pancakes warm; they are best when eaten fresh off the griddle and still warm.

Snack:
Whatever Snack You Want

The seventh day is your cheat day and you can have anything you want, but don't go overboard. Just have a serving of it. This could be French fries, a donut, a slice of cake, or whatever you desire.

I suggest buying your cheat snack rather than making it at home, otherwise you will bring unwanted ingredients and food into your home and mess up your diet. Furthermore, it will be an added burden to clean your pantry and refrigerator of unhealthy food once again.

Lunch:
The Best Steak Salad

To make the best steak salad, you need to cook the best steak, and that's really easy.

*   Season your steak well. Cook the steak in a blazing hot pan. If you have a cast iron pan, use it and don't put the steak in the pan until it's smoking like mad. This high heat is what gives the steak a gorgeous char without overcooking it.

*   Since you're using such high heat, oil the steak instead of the pan. Make sure the steak you buy is at least 3/4 inch thick. The more thick of a steak, the better.

- If you salt your steak well and cook it quickly over super high heat, you'll have the best steak ever for your steak salad.

 Tips

- ✓ Arugula, try baby greens or crunchy romaine
- ✓ Cucumbers, try celery or bell peppers
- ✓ Tomatoes, try mangos or persimmons
- ✓ Red onion, try radishes

Ingredients:

The steak:

- 1 10-ounce grilling steak (boneless prime rib)
- 1/2 teaspoon each salt and pepper
- 1 teaspoon avocado oil

The salad:

- 4 ounces of arugula
- 1 cup cherry tomatoes, cut in half
- 1/2 English cucumber, diced
- 1/2 avocado, sliced
- 1/4 cup thinly sliced red onions

Creamy balsamic dressing:

- 1/2 tablespoon each: grainy mustard, Dijon mustard, and balsamic vinegar
- 2 tablespoons olive oil
- A pinch of salt and pepper

Directions:

1. Take the steak out of your refrigerator and evenly coat both the sides with salt and pepper. Add all the salad ingredients to a salad bowl.

2. Heat a cast iron or heavy bottomed pan over high heat. Drizzle the avocado oil over both sides of the steak. When the pan starts to smoke, add the steak and let it cook undisturbed for 2 minutes. Flip the steak over and let it cook for 2-3 minutes more. Transfer the steak to a cutting board and let it rest.

3. Whisk the salad dressing ingredients in a small bowl. Thin the dressing with up to a tablespoon of water, as needed. Pour the dressing over the salad and toss.

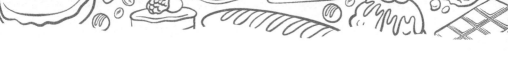

4. Thinly slice the steak across the grain and serve it over the salad.

The salad dressing will keep for a few weeks in your refrigerator, so feel free to make extra to have on hand for your dinner salads.

 Dinner:
Deviled Chicken

Ingredients:

- 6 chicken leg quarters
- 1/4 cup butter, melted
- 1 tablespoon lemon juice
- 1 tablespoon prepared mustard
- 1 teaspoon salt
- 1 teaspoon paprika
- 1/4 teaspoon pepper

Directions:

1. Preheat the oven to 375° F. Place chicken in a 15x10x1-in. baking pan. In a small bowl, combine the remaining ingredients and pour over chicken.
2. Bake uncovered for 50-60 minutes or until a thermometer reads 170°-175° F, basting occasionally with pan juices.

 # Chapter Summary

✓ After the first three days of going without sugar completely, you'll experience sugar cravings and withdrawal symptoms.

✓ To take care of these, it's time to incorporate fruits in your diet after three days; but do this slowly. Fruits have natural sugar that satisfy your cravings, ease the withdrawal symptoms, and don't mess up your sugar detox journey.

✓ Eating fruits as such may sound boring to some. Therefore, I've given a few recipes with fruits to try out and get the maximum nourishment in a delicious way.

Okay, so you've successfully completed a week of the sugar detox! Kudos to you and your willpower. Only the final 3 days are left now, so don't give up!

When you feel things getting challenging or you want to give up, remember the reason you started on this journey. You might need help from your supportive community you've built to stay on track for your health goals.

It won't serve you to give up when you are so near to achieving your goals! So, get ready to savor the final three days of your journey with the following recipes.

DAY 08

Breakfast:
Almond Butter Blueberry Waffles

These waffles are golden and crispy on the outside.

Ingredients:

- 2/3 cup natural creamy almond butter
- 2 eggs
- 1/2 banana, mashed
- 1/4 teaspoon almond extract
- 1/2 tablespoon coconut oil, melted and cooled
- 1/3 cup unsweetened almond milk
- 1 tablespoon coconut flour
- 1/2 teaspoon baking soda
- 1 teaspoon cinnamon
- 1/8 teaspoon salt (only if your almond butter is not salted)
- 2/3 cup fresh or frozen blueberries

Directions:

1. Preheat the waffle iron and spray with nonstick cooking spray. Whisk together almond butter, eggs, banana, almond extract, coconut oil, and almond milk in a large bowl until there aren't any lumps.

2. Add coconut flour, baking soda, cinnamon, and salt to this batter. Mix well. Gently fold in blueberries.

3. Put a spoonful of batter into waffle iron and cook until the steam stops, and waffles are golden brown and crispy on the outside. Repeat with the remaining batter.

4. Serve immediately.

Snack:

Lavender Blueberry Smoothie with Cauliflower

In this recipe, cauliflower and zucchini are used as a base for the smoothie. Cauliflower gives your smoothie it's creamy texture similar to bananas, but without the sugar. Lightly steam the vegetable before blending to make it easier on your digestion.

Zucchinis also provides a creamy texture to the smoothie, but it won't overpower you in flavor and blends well with the other fruits and vegetables. It's also important to lightly steam it for easier digestibility. Blueberries and lavender leaves add so much flavor to your smoothie. Blueberries are a low-glycemic fruit and full of antioxidants. Lavender leaves not only add flavor, but also help calm your mind.

Almond milk is the liquid used in this recipe, but you can also try hemp, cashew, macadamia, or coconut milk. Nut butter is a healthy fat, and flax seeds are a superfood. They are full of fiber and are a good source of micronutrients like iron, chromium, cobalt, manganese, selenium, zinc, copper, and iodine. Dates provide a nice punch of sweetness to your smoothie, but they are completely optional.

Ingredients:

- 1 cup cauliflower (lightly steamed, then frozen)
- 1/2 cup zucchini (lightly steamed, then frozen)
- 1/4 cup frozen blueberries
- 1 tsp. dried lavender leaves or 1-2 fresh flowers
- 1-2 dates (optional)
- 1 tsp. nut butter
- 1 tsp. ground flax

- 1 packet of Vanilla Daily Shake
- 1/4 tsp. cinnamon
- 1/4 tsp. vanilla powder
- 3/4 – 1 cup almond milk
- 1 tsp. lemon juice (optional)

Directions:

1. Add all the ingredients to a blender and blend till you get a smoothie that is creamy and thick.
2. If you like your smoothies on the thinner side, add more liquid to it and blend well.
3. Pour into a glass or a bowl and top with blueberries, millet puffs, edible flowers, and coconut shavings.
4. Enjoy your smoothie.

Lunch:
Creamy Garlic Mushroom Chicken

This recipe is high in protein and low in carbs. I used mushrooms, as they are low in calories and naturally high in protein, Vitamin C, and iron. However, if you don't like mushrooms, you can use spinach instead. Add a touch of parmesan to snazz it up to have a Creamy Garlic Spinach Chicken.

For this recipe, have your chicken ready. Portion it out into 4 pieces, defrost it in the microwave or with hot water, and flatten it out between two sheets of baking paper with either a meat mallet, the heel of your hand, or the bottom of any jar.

Ingredients:

- 1 lb. chicken
- 3 tbsp. cream
- 3 tbsp. chicken stock
- A pinch of salt
- 1 cup button mushrooms, diced
- 1 tsp.. butter
- 1-2 tbsp. crushed garlic
- 1/3 cup Shallots, sliced
- 1 teaspoon Cornflour/Cornstarch
- 1/2 teaspoon Lemon juice, optional

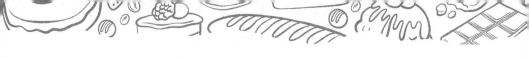

- 240 grams brown lentils tinned
- 1 cup Frozen mix (Peas/Corn/Carrot)
- 1 teaspoon Oregano dried
- 1 teaspoon Thyme dried

Directions:

1. Flatten out the chicken using a meat mallet or the heel of your hand.
2. Cook the chicken pieces in a pan on medium to high heat for about 4 minutes on each side until golden brown.
3. Remove the cooked chicken pieces from the pan and place in an oven to keep warm.
4. Place the tinned lentils, frozen veggie mix, stock, and dried herbs into a separate saucepan on low heat for 5 minutes, and prepare the mushroom sauce in the meantime.
5. In the same pan you cooked the chicken, add a teaspoon of butter, garlic, shallots, and diced mushrooms. Toss about for a few minutes until cooked.
6. Add the lemon juice, chicken broth, cream, and salt. Stir to form a sauce like consistency.
7. To thicken the sauce, take a tablespoon of liquid from the pan, mix it with the cornflour, and add it back into the sauce. Stir to thicken.
8. Place the chicken onto the lentil mix, and drizzle the creamy mushroom sauce over it. Garnish with additional chopped shallots.

Dinner:

Cajun Shrimp and Rice

Ingredients:

- 1 tablespoon olive oil
- 1 tablespoon butter
- 1 yellow onion, diced
- 2 stalks celery, diced
- 1 green bell pepper, seeded and diced
- 2 cloves garlic, minced
- 2 teaspoons paprika
- 1/2 teaspoon dried oregano
- 1/2 teaspoon dried thyme
- 1/4 teaspoon cayenne pepper

- 1/4 teaspoon crushed red pepper flakes
- 1 cup uncooked white rice
- 2 cups vegetable broth
- 1 pound shrimp, peeled and deveined
- 1 tablespoon lemon juice

Directions:

1. Heat oil and butter in a medium pot over medium heat.
2. Add onion, celery, and bell pepper. Sauté for 4-5 minutes until they become soft.
3. Add garlic, paprika, oregano, thyme, cayenne pepper, and crushed red pepper flakes. Cook for another one minute till fragrant.
4. Add brown rice and broth. Season with salt and pepper as per your taste.
5. Increase the heat to high and bring the mixture to a boil. Reduce the heat to low, cover, and cook for about 10 minutes or till most of the liquid is absorbed and rice is evenly cooked.
6. Add in the shrimp. Cover and cook for about five minutes until shrimp is pink and opaque. Top it with lemon juice and serve.

DAY 09

Breakfast:
Breakfast Fried Brown Rice

Ingredients:

- 1 cup cooked brown rice, preferably leftover from the day before
- 6 slices thick-cut bacon, chopped.
  - Try to find bacon without added nitrates. Can be found at any healthy food store
- 2 large eggs, lightly beaten
- 1 to 2 teaspoons low-sodium soy sauce
- 4 green onions, sliced
- 2 teaspoons toasted sesame oil
- **For serving:**
  - 2 eggs, cooked as desired
  - 1/2 avocado, sliced
  - 1 tablespoon freshly snipped chives
  - Hot sauce

The Fastest & Easiest Way To Detox & Eliminate Sugar
In Only 10 Days To Lose Weight And Burn Fat

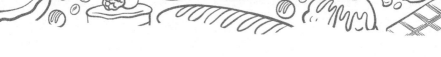

Directions:

1. Heat a large skillet or wok over low heat and add the bacon. Cook until its fat is rendered and bacon turns crispy. Remove it with a slotted spoon and place it on a paper towel to drain the extra grease.

2. Remove the bacon fat from the skillet in a bowl for later use. Leave about 1 tablespoon of fat in the skillet and heat it over medium-low heat.

3. Add eggs and constantly stir with a wooden spoon until the eggs are just scrambled. Remove them from flame and set aside.

4. Pour the remaining bacon fat in the skillet and increase the flame to high. Add in the rice, ross to coat well, and cook for 1-2 minutes.

5. Stir, breaking apart any pieces, and cook for another 1-2 minutes. Repeat till it gets golden brown and crispy.

6. At this point, taste the rice to check the seasoning, and add soy sauce. Add the bacon and eggs back into the skillet along with green onions.

7. Stir well and cook over low heat.

8. Cook the eggs as desired and season them with salt, pepper, and crushed red pepper.

9. Take out the rice in a bowl or a plate, and add the egg on top with a slice of avocado. Finish with a sprinkle of chives and enjoy.

 ### Snack:
Beet Hummus

This recipe amplifies the natural sweetness of beet during the roasting process. Beets contain folate which strengthens your immune system and prevents anemia. Manganese is the trace mineral found in beets that serve your immune system. Other micronutrients and antioxidants in beets assist in keeping common colds at bay.

Garlic is used in this recipe not only for flavor, but its antibacterial and antiviral properties. Olive oil is known for increasing the lifespan, slowing the ageing process, preventing heart disease, and aiding in weight loss.

Ingredients:

*   1 large beet or a few small (about 1 1/2 cups, peeled and chopped)
*   15.5-ounce can of garbanzo beans
*   1/3 cup olive oil
*   2-4 cloves garlic
*   1 lemon

- Salt, to taste
- Pepper, to taste
- Cayenne pepper, to taste

Directions:

1. Preheat the oven to 400° F. Peel the beets and cut them into large chunks.
2. Spread them on a baking sheet. Drizzle with olive oil, salt, and cayenne pepper. Bake the beets for 25-35 minutes, occasionally stirring in between and checking if cooked. When done, beets should be easily pierced by a fork.
3. Cool the beets to room temperature and prepare other ingredients.
4. Strain and rinse the garbanzo beans. Zest lemon. Peel the garlic. Place all the ingredients with beets in a food processor.
5. Blend until the mixture is smooth and fully combined.
6. Serve immediately or store in the refrigerator for a week. Drizzle some olive oil over the top while serving.

Lunch:
Kale Quinoa and Avocado Salad

Ingredients:

Salad:

- 2/3 cup quinoa
- 11/3 cups water
- 1 bunch kale, torn into bite-sized pieces
- 1/2 avocado - peeled, pitted, and diced
- 1/2 cup chopped cucumber
- 1/3 cup chopped red bell pepper
- 2 tablespoons chopped red onion
- 1 tablespoon crumbled feta cheese

Dressing:

- 1/4 cup olive oil
- 2 tablespoons lemon juice
- 11/2 tablespoons Dijon mustard
- 3/4 teaspoon sea salt
- 1/4 teaspoon ground black pepper

Directions:

1. Boil quinoa with 1 1/3 cup of water in a saucepan. Reduce the heat to medium/low, cover, and cook till the water is absorbed and quinoa are tender (about 10-15 minutes). Set aside to cool.

2. Place kale in a steamer basket over 1 inch of boiling water in a saucepan. Cover and steam the kale until hot. Transfer it to a large plate.

3. Top it with quinoa, avocado, cucumber, bell pepper, red onion, and feta cheese.

4. Whisk olive oil, lemon juice, Dijon mustard, sea salt, and black pepper in a bowl until the oil emulsifies into a dressing. Pour over the salad and enjoy.

Dinner:
Grilled Basil Chicken and Tomatoes

Ingredients:

- 3/4 cup balsamic vinegar
- 1/4 cup tightly packed fresh basil leaves
- 2 tablespoons olive oil
- 1 clove garlic, minced
- 1/2 teaspoon salt
- 8 plum tomatoes
- 4 boneless, skinless, chicken breast halves (4 ounces each)

Directions:

1. Place the first 5 ingredients in a blender. Cut four tomatoes into quarters and add to the blender. Cover and process till blended well.

2. Halve the remaining tomatoes for grilling.

3. Combine chicken and 2/3 cup of the above marinade in a bowl. Refrigerate it for 1 hour, covered, turning occasionally. Keep the remaining marinade for serving.

4. After 1 hour, place chicken on an oil-grilled rack over medium heat. Discard the marinade left in the bowl. Grill the chicken, covered for 4-6 minutes on each side. Grill tomatoes, covered, over medium heat until light brown.

5. Serve chicken and tomatoes with the reserved marinade.

Breakfast:
Wheat Free Avocado Toast

I created this grain-free, vegan, soy-free cauliflower bread for this recipe.

Ingredients:

- 1 pound cauliflower florets
- 3 tablespoons ground chia seeds
- 3 tablespoons water
- 1/2 cup almond meal
- Large pinch of Himalayan salt
- 1 avocado
- Large handful arugula, washed
- 1/8 red onion, thinly sliced
- Optional: olive oil, lemon juice, garlic salt, Himalayan salt to top

Directions:

1. Preheat the oven to 400° F and line the baking sheet with parchment paper.
2. Place the cauliflower florets in a food processor and blend until you get a rice-like texture.
3. Pour the mixture into a large pot, add water, and bring to a boil. Cover, reduce the heat, and cook for about 5 minutes.
4. Drain the liquid and allow the cauliflower to cool for a few minutes.
5. Mix 2 tablespoons of ground chia with 3 tablespoons of water, and allow the mixture to thicken.
6. Once the cauliflower has cooled, transfer it into a nut milk bag or the thinnest dish towel or into a few paper towels. Squeeze the cauliflower to drain all the excess liquid.
7. Place the cauliflower in a large bowl, add chia, almond meal, and salt until the mixture forms a well-kneaded dough.
8. Press the dough into the parchment-lined baking sheet, keeping the crust about 1/4-inch thick. Bake at 400° F for 30 minutes, until the top is lightly golden and dry to touch.
9. Remove the bread from the oven. Using an additional piece of parchment paper and sheet pan, flip the bread over and bake for another 15 minutes.
10. Remove the bread from the oven and allow it to cool.

11. Mash the avocado with a pinch of Himalayan salt. Cut the cauliflower bread into 4 pieces, spread with a generous serving of avocado, and top with arugula and red onion.

12. Add any additional topping of your choice—another pinch of salt, a drizzle of olive oil and a squeeze of lemon to top it up. Enjoy your toast.

Snack:
Creamy Orange Coconut Smoothie Bowl

Ingredients:

- 1/4 cup unsweetened coconut milk
- 1/4 cup unsweetened vanilla coconut milk yogurt
- 1 teaspoon vanilla extract
- 1/2 frozen banana
- 1 1/2 peeled, seedless mandarin orange, divided
- Ice, as desired
- 2 tablespoons pistachios
- 2 tablespoons dried shredded coconut
- 2 tablespoons chia seeds

Directions:

1. Blend coconut milk, yogurt, vanilla, banana, 1 orange, and ice as desired.

2. Pour into a bowl, and top with remaining orange wedges, pistachios, coconut, and chia seeds. Enjoy your snack.

Lunch:
Garlic Ginger Shrimp with Quinoa and Tomato Salsa

Ingredients:

The Shrimp:

- 1/2 lb (200g) shrimp, raw, peeled and deveined
- 1 cup uncooked quinoa
- 1 tablespoon extra-virgin olive oil
- 1 teaspoon minced garlic
- 1 knob fresh ginger, minced
- 1 teaspoon cumin
- 1 pinch of cayenne pepper, optional (or any hot sauce you like)

- 1/4 cup lime juice
- Fresh cracked pepper, to taste

The salsa:

- A handful cherry tomatoes, diced
- 1 jalapeño, diced
- 1/2 red onion, finely minced
- 1/4 cup freshly chopped cilantro

The sauce:

- 3 tablespoons Greek yogurt
- 2 tablespoons olive oil
- 1 pinch cumin
- Salt and fresh cracked black pepper

Directions:

1. Prepare quinoa as directed on its packet and set aside.
2. Combine the salsa ingredients in a salad bowl and set aside.
3. Heat olive oil in a medium skillet, add garlic and ginger. Sauté for 2 minutes. Add shrimp, cumin, and cayenne pepper, and cook for 3 minutes on each side till cooked through. Season with black pepper and add lime juice. Remove from the skillet and set aside.
4. To prepare the dressing, whisk lime juice, Greek yogurt, olive oil, cumin, salt, and pepper.
5. In a meal plate, place the shrimp, quinoa, and salsa. Drizzle the dressing on the top and enjoy.

Dinner:
Cumin Chili Spiced Flank Steak

Ingredients:

- 2 small red peppers, cut into 2-inch strips
- 1 small yellow pepper, cut into 2-inch strips
- 2 cups grape tomatoes
- 1 small onion, cut into 1/2-inch wedges
- 2 jalapeno peppers, halved and seeded
- 2 tablespoons olive oil, divided
- 3/4 teaspoon salt, divided

The Fastest & Easiest Way To Detox & Eliminate Sugar
In Only 10 Days To Lose Weight And Burn Fat

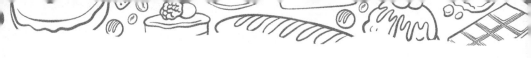

- 3/4 teaspoon pepper, divided
- 2 teaspoons ground cumin
- 1 teaspoon chili powder
- 1 beef flank steak
- 2-3 teaspoons lime juice
- Hot cooked couscous
- Lime wedges

Directions:

1. Preheat a boiler. Place the first 5 ingredients in a greased 15x10x1-in. baking pan. Toss with 1 tablespoon olive oil, ¼ teaspoon salt and ¼ teaspoon pepper. Cook for 10-12 minutes or until vegetables are tender and begin to char, turning once.

2. Mix salt, pepper, cumin, chili powder and the remaining oil. Rub it over both sides of the steak. Grill, covered, over medium heat or broil 4 in. from heat, 6-9 minutes on each side. Let it stand for 5 minutes.

3. For salsa, chop broiled onion and jalapenos, and place in a small bowl. Stir in tomatoes and lime juice. Thinly slice the steak across the grain. Serve with salsa, broiled peppers, couscous and lime wedges.

> ⚠️ **WARNING:** Wear disposable gloves while handling hot peppers to avoid skin burns. Avoid touching your face during and after the task.

 Bonus Recipes

You'll find these recipes useful to spice up your regular meals.

Homemade Hot sauce

Ingredients:

- 20 habanero peppers (4.5 ounces)
- 5 serrano peppers (2.5 ounces)
- 15 dried arbol chiles
- 2 large carrots (5.5 ounces), peeled, halved lengthwise and quartered
- 1 large sweet onion (15 ounces), cut into eight wedges
- 8 garlic cloves, halved
- 1 cup water

- 3/4 cup high-quality white vinegar (minimum 5% acetic acid)
- 1/2 cup fresh lime juice
- 3 teaspoons salt
- 1 teaspoon coarsely ground pepper

Directions:

1. Cut habanero and serrano peppers into half. Discard the stem and the seeds saving just the flesh. Cover the arbol chiles with boiling water and keep them aside to rehydrate for 10 minutes.
2. Once softened, strain out the chilies and discard the water. Always wear gloves when handling hot peppers.
3. Fill a 6-quart stockpot with a gallon of water and bring it to a boil. Add the carrots, onions, and garlic, and simmer until soft. Remove the vegetables to a bowl with a slotted spoon.
4. Add the peppers to the stockpot and return the mixture to a boil. Boil for 1 minute before removing the peppers to the vegetable bowl. Discard any remaining water.
5. Place the cooked vegetables and chilies in a blender. Add water, vinegar, lime juice, salt, and pepper to the blender. Puree until the mixture is very smooth.
6. Bring the mixture to a boil over medium-high heat. Remove the pot from the flame and set it aside.
7. Prepare five half-pint jars by sanitizing them according to the package directions. Carefully pour the boiled hot sauce into the half-pint jars, leaving 1/2-inch headspace at the top. Remove the air bubbles, and adjust the headspace, if necessary, by adding additional hot sauce.
8. Wipe the rims clean and close the jars. Screw the lids on until they are fingertip tight.
9. Place the jars into a canner with simmering water until they are completely submerged and covered with water. Bring the canner to a boil and process for 10 minutes. Carefully remove the jars from the canner and allow them to cool at room temperature.
10. Enjoy your hot sauce with a variety of dishes.

Easy Kimchi

Kimchi is a traditional Korean dish made by fermenting cabbage, red pepper, and other vegetables. It's full of probiotics taking care of your digestion and overall health. Fermentation keeps micronutrients and antioxidant levels of the vegetables intact, and promotes the development of healthy bacteria in the gut. These bacteria help fight infection, improve immunity, and enhance the body's ability to produce vitamins.

Cabbage, the star of Kimchi, has 35 different antioxidants, fiber, potassium, Vitamin A, B, and C, magnesium, and calcium. Regular consumption of cabbage lowers the risk of heart disease and type 2 diabetes.

Green onions, being rich in Vitamin C and K are used in the recipe, and are a great choice for optimal bone health.

Ingredients:

- 2 lb. napa cabbage
- 3-5 green onions
- 1/2 tablespoon ginger
- 1 tablespoon garlic
- 3-6 tablespoons Korean red pepper
- 2 tablespoons fish sauce
- 1 tablespoon water
- Salt

Directions:

1. Wash and cut the cabbage into bite-sized pieces. Place it in a large bowl, add a handful of salt and massage into the cabbage.
2. Cover the cabbage with water till fully submerged. Cover and let it sit for 24 hours.
3. Mix ginger, garlic, red pepper, coconut palm sugar, fish sauce, and water to make a paste. For a more spicier version, you can add up to 6 tablespoons of Korean red pepper.
4. After 24 hours soaking, drain and rinse the cabbage. Toss it with the spices paste and massage thoroughly.
5. Pack the cabbage mixture in a large, disinfected jar. Cover with an airtight lid and store in a dark, cool place for 24-72 hours for fermentation.
6. When done fermenting, store it in the refrigerator for about 3 weeks. Kimchi is safe beyond this period as well but the flavor will change slightly, and will be more enjoyable with cooked dishes like fried rice, rather than eating alone.

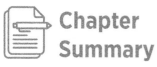

Chapter Summary

✓ Only the final 3 days remain on your sugar detox journey and you have been doing well. Don't give up!

✓ Moreover, it won't serve you to give up when you are so near to achieving your health goals and transforming your eating habits.

✓ When things seem challenging, remember the reason you started on this journey and take help from your supportive community.

The 30-Day Detox And Beyond

Congratulations on completing the first 10 days of sugar detox!

These 10 days are crucial in readjusting your palate and eating habits. Your cravings for sugar should have subsided by now. If you are able to make it past the first 10 days, it gets a lot easier to do another 10 days, then another, and then another. That means you will be on your way to continuing this lifestyle for 20 days, 30 days, or maybe even 6 months to a year more!

Once this happens, leading a healthy lifestyle becomes second nature. You will have a lifestyle of true freedom from wanting or needing sugar all the time, and retraining your palate to taste the natural sweetness in things and ways you never did before!

So, what are the top 10 benefits of living sugar free?

Top 10 Benefits of Living Sugar-Free

1. You start appreciating fruits for their color and naturally sweet taste.
2. Your taste buds become more sensitive now. Things which tasted plain to you will taste sweeter now.
3. You get to discover and explore a variety of whole and packaged foods you didn't even know about before, like avocado toasts, Greek yogurt, etc.
4. You start losing those extra pounds. This can be one of the motivating factors to keep you on track of this journey.
5. The most visible side-effect of going sugar-free is losing your belly fat.
6. You start feeling fresher, healthier, and more vibrant when you wake up in the morning, free from the regrets of eating any unhealthy food the day before.
7. You feel good and positive about yourself and wish to continue in an upward spiral towards a healthy lifestyle.
8. Your decision-making skills and food choices get a lot better and improve.
9. You understand food and nutrition for your body in a much better way, such as how sugar harms your body, and what are the best alternatives for your health.
10. You are more mentally and emotionally sound than ever before.

Now that you know the benefits, it shouldn't be a dilemma anymore on how to continue in your future of eating more whole foods, no refined sugar, and leaving a room for that dessert on only special occasions.

What foods can you actually eat?

An average American adult consumes about 82 grams or 26 teaspoons of added sugar in a day, on top of the naturally occurring sugars consumed through fruits, grains, and milk products.

However, excessive sugar consumption poses a risk for:

- Obesity
- Diabetes
- Heart disease
- Increased inflammation in the body
- High cholesterol
- High blood pressure

You can significantly reduce the risk of these diseases by adopting a no-sugar diet plan. So, here are a few tips on how to get started, foods to look out for, and sweet substitutes to try.

Start Gradually

There's no point in making an eating plan you can't stick to. Therefore, take the plunge slowly. Take the first few weeks as a period of lower sugar rather than no sugar. Your palate and taste buds will readjust to the less-sugary lifestyle, and eventually you won't crave high-sugar foods the way you did before.

During this time, eat foods with natural sugars like fruits, as they are packed with nutrients and fiber. Other ways to decrease the intake of sugar are:

- Put less sweetener in your tea, coffee, or breakfast cereal.
- Swap regular sodas and fruit juices with flavored carbonated water that is devoid of artificial sweeteners. Or infuse water with your favorite fruit.
- Go for unflavored yogurt instead of a full-flavored pack. Try flavoring your plain yogurt with berries.
- Watch the amount of dried fruit you eat, as it normally has added sugar on top of its high sugar content. Replace them with fresh berries.

The Fastest & Easiest Way To Detox & Eliminate Sugar
In Only 10 Days To Lose Weight And Burn Fat

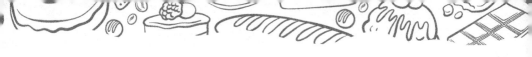

- Choose to eat grains with no added sugar. Read food labels to make sure you're not getting added sugar in foods.

These small changes are easy to incorporate, will keep your cravings and withdrawal symptoms in check, and put you closer on the path to success in your health goals. Although, if you have a severe addiction to sugar, then you should just cut it out all at once.

Dump the Obvious Sources of Sugar

These include:

➡ Breakfast pastries, like muffins and coffee cake

➡ Baked goods, like cookies and cake

➡ Frozen treats, like ice cream and sorbet

Also, remove foods high in naturally occurring sugar like:

➡ Dried fruits, like dates and raisins

➡ Yogurt with added fruit or other flavors

➡ Milk

➡ Honey and maple syrup

Start Reading Food Labels

There's hidden sugar found in many products in your grocery stores, such as:

➡ Baked beans

➡ Crackers

➡ Tacos

➡ Boxed rice

➡ Frozen entrees

➡ Grains, like bread, rice, and pasta

The simplest way to eliminate the hidden sources of sugar is to read the nutritional information and ingredients list found on the food label.

Keep in mind:

- Sugar is often measured in grams on labels. Four grams is equivalent to one teaspoon.
- Fruits don't come with an ingredients label, so you'll have to look up their nutritional information online.
- Nutrition labels have additional information to help you make informed decisions. They list both total sugars and added sugars.

Reading these food labels can be confusing, so download shopping apps on your phone that reveal your food facts on the go.

Learn the Different Names of Sugar

As we discussed in the previous chapters, "sugar" is known by 56 different names. You'll need to learn them all to completely remove it from your diet. As a general thumb rule, look out for ingredients ending in "-ose". These are usually forms of sugar.

Avoid Artificial Sweeteners

Artificial sweeteners are 200-13000 times sweeter than real sugar. In the long run, they trigger your sugar cravings making it harder for you to stick to your diet plan. Common sugar substitutes include:

➦ Splenda

➦ Equal

➦ Sweet 'N Low

➦ NutraSweet

These sugar substitutes are usually found in products marketed as low-sugar, no-sugar or low-calorie.

Avoid Drinking Sugar

Sugar is also found in:

- Soda
- Fruit juices
- Flavored coffee

The Fastest & Easiest Way To Detox & Eliminate Sugar
In Only 10 Days To Lose Weight And Burn Fat

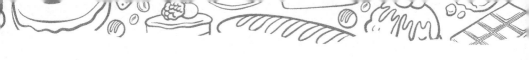

- Flavored milk
- Flavored tea
- Hot chocolate
- Tonic water
- Wine
- Cocktails
- After-dinner liquors

It's not only what you eat, but also what you drink that matters.

Opt for the Unsweetened Versions

Many foods and drinks come in sweetened and unsweetened varieties. Unsweetened versions usually don't have added sugars, but naturally occurring sugars may still be present. Therefore, read your food labels thoroughly before making the final selection.

Add More Flavor Without Adding Sugar

Eliminating sugar doesn't mean eating food that's bland. Look for spices, condiments, seasonings, and other natural things to add variety to your meals. For example, you can drop a cinnamon stick into your coffee cup or add the spice to your bowl of unflavored yogurt. Vanilla extract can also add a delicious flavor to your food without adding sugar.

Get Enough Nutrients from Other Sources

When eliminating foods laden with high sugar, it's mandatory to consume other foods that provide the right balance of nutrients. For example, if you eliminate fruits, vegetables can serve as an easy replacement for your fruit servings. Eat a variety of vegetables to ensure you get a full spectrum of nutrients.

Get Enough Nutrients from Other Sources

It's not easy to fully eliminate natural and added sugars. For some, the thought of never eating that piece of birthday cake may seem overwhelming and bring tears to their eyes. However, the truth is that total abstinence is not required.

You can limit your added sugar intake to nine teaspoons per day for men and six teaspoons per day for women, as recommended by the American Heart Association.

Once you retrain your palate through this journey, your desire for extra sweet foods won't be as strong. When adding sugar back in your diet, start with naturally occurring sugars, like fruits. You will find these will taste sweeter, and they'll be more satisfying once you have gone through the sugar elimination process.

Think of sugar like your favorite holiday—knowing that there's a sugary occasion to work toward may help you stick to your goals. On set occasions, you can fully savor the sugary food and then tuck away until the next time.

I know that going completely sugar free is not for everyone. You can limit the sugar for a short period of time, but it's difficult to leave it all together. Therefore, I recommend you alternate your no-sugar diet with a low-sugar diet from week to week, or you can replace refined sugars with naturally occurring sugar and reintroduce it in your diet slowly.

Whatever way you choose, you will definitely reap its health benefits if you stick to it. This way of eating will clear up your skin, increase your energy levels, and reduce those extra kilos you've been carrying. Further, these benefits keep on increasing over the long term.

So, finally you started with your sugar detox journey and successfully completed the first 10 days. What's next?

10-Day Sugar Detox Assessment

While starting on this journey, you took an assessment of your physical health to know where you stood at the moment. Ten days down the line, it's time to take another assessment, record your results, and note any healthy improvements you have experienced.

But what if you don't see any improvements? Relax! Continue to do 10 days of detox again and again until you start seeing improvements. Assess your health again after every 10 days.

First, note down the following:

- **Date:**
- **Weight:**
- **Waistline:**

The Fastest & Easiest Way To Detox & Eliminate Sugar
In Only 10 Days To Lose Weight And Burn Fat

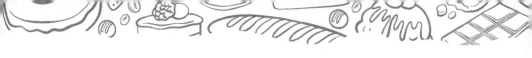

Next, comes the cognitive assessment results. Check all the following unhealthy symptoms you have or had:

- Anxiety
- Chronic Fatigue, Fibromyalgia
- Decreased Sex Drive
- Depression
- Fatigue
- Foggy Brained
- Food Allergies
- Insomnia
- Irritability
- Hormonal Imbalance
- Poor Memory
- Craving for sweets and refined carbohydrates or alcohol
- Digestive issues (bloating, constipation, diarrhea) or disorders
- Skin and nail infections such as toenail fungus, athlete's foot, and ringworm
- Vaginal yeast infections, urinary tract infections

Now, answer the following questions about yourself:

- Since you've reduced the amount of sugar or dense carbohydrates you've been eating, how do you feel now?

  _____

  _____

- How is your sleep? What about your digestive function?

  _____

  _____

- Do you think that eating high-calorie and high-sugar foods will make you feel better or worse?

  _____

  _____

- Has the time and energy commitment that's gone into avoiding sugar and dense carbs added more stress to your life? How much sugar or carbs have controlled your life and food choices?

_____

_____

Important Things to Remember

Those who began this sugar detox for the first time, it must have been a HUGE change in your dietary habits. If you've been eating bread, cereals, and pasta on a regular basis, this detox was essentially an elimination diet for you. Because of this, you need to go slow on reintroducing foods like wheat, soy, and dairy.

Consider how often you consume sweetened or high-carb foods, and then decide whether or not to add some of those foods back into your diet, perhaps once-a-day versus at every meal would be a healthier option for you on a regular basis.

Ponder whether you previously ate sweets or dense carbs as a reward, comfort, or just out of habit. Check whether or not eating such foods made you feel your best or helped you reach your health goals.

Now, health goals could be varied. Every person could have different health goals. A lot of people lose weight during this detox journey; however, that might not be the primary goal of yours.

If you lost weight, recognize the fact that a bite of sweets here and there that seemed innocent enough was actually too much for you or your health goals. Even if your primary goal was not to lose weight but to break away from the unhealthy eating habits and conquer your cravings, think if you start eating sweets again, will it trigger your problems or not? Will it lead to a downward spiral in your health goals? And then, consciously watch and choose what you eat on a daily basis.

To safely and slowly add naturally occurring sugars and starches to your diet, consider the portions you eat and the time you eat them.

- If you had issues with your blood sugar regulation previously, don't consume fruits alone.
- Fruit consumption also depends on your activity level. Eat small portions of berries or half a piece of fruit if you aren't very active, or larger portions if you are active.
- Starchy foods must be added back on days when you are most active, and

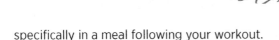

specifically in a meal following your workout.

- If you aren't very active physically, keep the portions of starchy foods to a minimum and don't allow them to rule your food plate, especially if you wish to lose weight and maintain it.

If you simply want to avoid your sugar cravings and you feel okay by not having them, you can enjoy root vegetables and tubers like sweet potatoes and squash more frequently. However, continue to avoid refined carbohydrates like bread, pasta, cereal, and other products made from flours, as well as packaged foods.

Never go on a sugar bend. Some of my clients, after completing their detox for the first time, went out and had candy following the day when they were hungry. When you are hungry, your blood sugar is already low, and by eating this candy, there's a sudden spike in your blood sugar which crashes in about an hour or two and makes you feel sleepy.

Even so, I am guilty of doing it. The first time I completed the detox, I ate candy the following day when I was hungry. I spiked my blood sugar so high that when it crashed about an hour or two later, I nearly passed out. Seriously, it was that intense. I vowed at that point that I'd never let that happen again.

Hopefully, you'll learn from my mistake too.

Take-Away Message

You can continue to live the no-sugar lifestyle until the end of time, but the majority of people (even me) who still enjoy a cake or ice-cream on occasions is absolutely fine.

I always advise my clients to follow the 80/20 rule after detox. The rule is to eat healthy, amazing foods for your body 80% of the time, and enjoying the foods you know are not the best for you for the rest 20% of the time.

This gives you some balance and freedom to enjoy life and not be entirely consumed by that sugar monster like before. In my personal experience, it is actually healthy to eat unhealthy foods sometimes. That's because if you eat healthy 100% of the time, you will crave that unhealthy food at some point of time. And ultimately, you will start binging and eating those unhealthy foods for months.

I have been through this situation before, and it is not great. Now I follow the 80/20 rule to keep myself in check and give myself a reward when I want to.

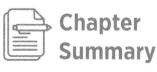

Chapter Summary

✓ The first 10 days of sugar detox retrains your palate and curbs your sugar cravings. Now, you won't crave sugar as much as you did before.

✓ It makes it easier for you to continue with this lifestyle in future.

✓ Going sugar-free helps you lose weight, belly fat, feel more positive about yourself, and make better food choices for yourself.

✓ To start with the sugar detox journey, take the plunge slowly by going a few weeks on lower sugar rather than no sugar.

✓ Assess your physical health after 10 days of sugar detox and record the changes you experience.

✓ It's practically not feasible to ditch sugar completely, especially when you love those cakes and ice-creams, so follow the 80/20 rule for your eating habits.

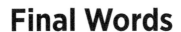

Final Words

By now, you know that 35% of the adult population in the United States has been diagnosed with pre-diabetic sugar levels. The cases of obesity, hypertension, high cholesterol, and heart disease are also increasing year by year.

You might be one of them, or you may land up with these diseases in future, especially if they run in your family.

The culprit of all these chronic diseases is none other than SUGAR! It's the root cause of all your skin problems—acne, rashes, eczema, and dandruff lead to more serious problems like diabetes, high blood pressure, high cholesterol, obesity, and a myriad of other health problems. Even after taking regular medications, these problems might not seem under control because you don't address the primary cause: THE SUGAR.

However, it's not easy to tackle with sugar. That's because the problem with sugar is ADDICTION. We all are obsessed with eating sugar despite knowing it's bad effects, making it difficult to control the urge. Each time we see a sweet snack, we can't stop ourselves from shoving it into our mouths. Our brains have been wired in that way that we seek high-calorie and sugary foods since the beginning of human evolution. Even our taste buds feel the sweet taste more than the salty or spicy tastes.

Moreover, sugar is now easily accessible in almost every food like bread, frozen ready-to-eat meals, candy, sodas, and pasta sauces. It's much cheaper than before. To add to the situation, we have a store counter located everywhere nowadays, loaded with chocolates, chips, and junk food. This junk food sells the most and stays on the market shelves longer.

Food scientists know about our sugar cravings and the addictive nature of sugar. Therefore, they manufacture products that appeal to our taste buds and market them in attention-grabbing colored bags to lure the public. Sugar is also cheaper than other items reducing the cost of production.

Sometimes, these high-calorie and sugary foods are also marketed under the name of "health products", having lots of proteins, low fat, or being gluten-free to fool the masses.

Also, if we don't have sugar for even a day, it can make us feel weak, lethargic, angry, moody, and down. We feel bloated and anxious, and savoring those syrupy snacks seems like a quick fix.

Even research studies have proven the addictive nature of sugar. Sugar, like any other drug of abuse—such as cocaine, morphine, or heroin—causes the release of dopamine and endorphins from our brain. These are feel-good chemicals and they give us a sense of pleasure. However, we need to consume sugar or drugs in ever increasing amounts to get the same amount of pleasure.

This means that if we consumed 2 teaspoons of sugar at one time, we need more than 2 teaspoons to get that same feel-good factor from it in the coming days.

But why is sugar so addictive?

Science says that a substance becomes addictive when it is refined. The problem is not with naturally occurring sugars, but with the refined sugar and refined carbohydrates we consume, like bread, pasta, cereals, dried fruit, etc. Sugar addiction also occurs when it is consumed in a binge-like manner. Bingeing is laying your hands on sugar or sweet snacks whenever you see them, regardless of whether you are hungry or not.

Refined sugar is derived from the natural sugarcane crop. However, the process of refinement concentrates the amount of sugar in the end product. This means sugar tastes sweeter than the same amount of sugarcane used to create it, and is highly addictive.

All addictive substances have health hazards, and so does sugar. Consuming it in high amounts messes with our hormones, and it results in increased production of insulin in our body, which leads to the storing of fat in our body cells. Thus, instead of burning fat, you'll be in a state of constantly storing it in your body and gaining weight.

A diet high in sugar is also linked to Alzheimer's, a progressive brain disorder that causes the brain cells to waste away and die. Sugar is also one of the leading causes of dementia, a continuous decline in thinking, behavioral and social skills that disrupt a person's ability to function independently.

The solution? A SUGAR DETOX! However, what matters is how you do it!

Going completely sugar-free for your whole life doesn't seem possible, right? Imagine a life without your favorite dessert!

The best way is to do the 10-day sugar detox, which I have covered in this book. I have guided you through the initial steps you should take to rid yourself of your sugar addiction in 10 days. These initial 10 days are the toughest because you'll have those sugar cravings and withdrawal symptoms weakening your willpower.

Luckily, I have guided you on how to stand strong and not let those cravings or withdrawal symptoms overpower you. That's why I always recommend you to take this plunge slowly. Start with a few weeks of lower sugar rather than no sugar, and then gradually ditch the unhealthy carbs and sweets you've been accustomed to.

Start your sugar detox journey by making a firm decision. Your decision is your commitment. Decide that you will switch to a healthier lifestyle. Decide that you will lose weight and lead a better quality of life. Decide to implement all the steps I detail in this book for the betterment of your health.

Making this decision is of prime importance, but what matters more is your ability to stick to it. Sticking to your decision and staying disciplined along the sugar detox gets easier once you understand how sugar addiction affects you physically and mentally, the types of food you should avoid and why, and what you'll gain by sugar detoxing.

Initially, you will start by dumping all forms of processed sugars for 10 days, and then extend it to 30 days to see the benefits it has on your health. Down the line, eating sugar-free foods will become the part and parcel of your lifestyle, and you won't go back to your old, unhealthy eating habits.

Dumping sugar doesn't mean getting rid of natural sugars, but avoiding processed sugars and refined carbohydrates which include rice, wheat, white bread, cereals, potato chips, sodas, and crackers. You'll be ditching all of these and consuming their healthier counterparts.

There are challenges many of you will face in going on a sugar-free diet. It will make you moody and angry. You'll feel that you can't eat to your satiety if you don't have sugar. Your brain will overpower you to eat more, no matter how much you ate before. No logic, no reasoning can stop you from biting into any snack you lay your hands on.

Therefore, I always recommend starting your journey with an assessment of your physical health. What's your weight, waistline, or do you have any symptoms of ill-health. Also, take an online cognitive test to determine the health of your brain.

It might sound that this sugar detox thing is for those with a chronic disease like diabetes, hypertension, skin problems, and others; but that's not true.

Anybody who wants to quit sugar and switch to a healthier lifestyle or want to control their eating habits and make better food choices can leverage from my sugar detox training detailed in this book.

It's quite possible that you don't have a full-fledged disease now, but you might have symptoms like anxiety, fatigue, mood swings, depression, foggy brain, food allergies, difficulty sleeping, poor memory, digestive problems, skin problems, etc. You probably never thought that the real cause of these symptoms can be an overconsumption of sugar.

So, take note of any such symptoms you have or experienced anytime in the past, and write a contract to yourself committing to ditch sugar and dense carbs along with the health goals you wish to achieve out of it.

After making a commitment to yourself, it's time to build a network of people who will support you thick and thin along this journey. Mind you, the sugar detox journey won't be easy. Though I have guided you at each step with my instructions and recommendations, you'll experience ups and downs along it. You'll have mood swings, withdrawal symptoms, cravings, and may feel like giving up.

This is the time when you'll need the help and motivation from your support system. Your support system should comprise people who share the same health goals as yours, and are willing to traverse the journey along with you. They must be good listeners and able to provide you with honest feedback on your actions.

To build your support system, start with people in your life—family, friends, neighbors, colleagues, co-workers, and/or social media friends. Make a list of people and divide them into positive and negative categories.

The positive category has people who are healthy, positive, and supportive of your health goals. Place people who are blamers, liars, critics, alcoholics, and drug abusers in a negative category. Such people will bog you down and drain your energy, so it's best to limit your contact with them during your health journey, otherwise they won't allow you to reach your goals.

Now, it's time to clear your house, pantry, and refrigerator of all unhealthy and unwanted food items like wheat, white flour, sugar, high fructose corn syrup, white rice, corn, milk products, soy products, artificial sweeteners, dried fruits, processed foods, vegetable oils, peanuts, margarine, canned food, sodas, fruit juices, diet drinks, and "low-fat" food. This is essential because if you have junk and high-sugar foods at home, your brain will drive you to eat them since they are more handy, and you'll relapse into your old eating habits.

It's simple to know if your food has a high sugar content or not. If it's not a plant, a protein or a healthy fat, don't buy it from the store or remove it from your house. Also, get into the habit of reading your food labels before you buy them.

Additionally, learn the 56 different names sugar is known by—dextrose, fructose, levulose, galactose, beet sugar, cane sugar, castor sugar, corn syrup solids, dextrin, ethyl maltol, icing sugar, maltodextrin, barley malt, caramel, golden syrup, honey, maple syrup, molasses, treacle, etc.

This is important because sugar is a substance of disguise. Many food manufacturers don't mention sugar on their manufactured products. They use a variety of names to trick you into buying them, so learning these names will be beneficial to you.

However, the major challenge in clearing your house of unhealthy food is a family member who wants to consume such type of food items. This may tempt you to eat as well, so tell that family member to keep these packets hidden in their room and out of the pantry or refrigerator.

After getting rid of all unwanted food items from your house, it's time to replace them with healthier options like meats, seafood, vegetables, low-glycemic fruits, nuts, seeds, legumes, beans, spices, whole grains, eggs, butter, and sugar-free protein powder.

Apart from eating healthy, you must ensure to drink the desired quantity of water in a day. Water is the most important nutrient for changing your lifestyle. If you don't consume adequate amounts of water daily, your body will suffer from dehydration, fatigue, constipation, dry mouth, dry skin, kidney problems, bladder problems and high blood pressure. Various sources recommend drinking half your weight (in pounds) in ounces of water every day. However, your daily requirement also depends on your activity levels.

Remember, drinking teas, juices, sodas, or other drinks don't hydrate your body adequately. They are not a replacement for water, as the majority of people think. They are diuretics, which cause you to urinate more and lose water from your body faster, thus making you more dehydrated.

During this sugar detox, you'll be eating differently than you ate before, so it's quite natural to feel cranky, irritable, and lethargic. To ease these withdrawal symptoms, you should cut out all sugars at once for three days, even the sugars from natural sources like fruits.

During these three days, keep yourself full and satisfied by consuming foods rich in fats like fish, nuts, and avocados. Eat lots of vegetables and organic protein to keep you feeling full and to keep your appetite under control.

After cutting out all sugar for three days, incorporate the natural sources of sugar like fruits in your diet, but slowly.

Going on a sugar detox doesn't mean you have to leave taste behind. Your food does not need to taste bland. Therefore, I have given you recipes for the 10-day sugar detox keeping in mind the foods you should consume and recipes that will taste amazing.

Most importantly, I don't believe in going sugar-free completely, so I have included a cheat day to enjoy the dessert of your choice once in these 10 days. I also advise you to keep those sugar treats for special occasions like family dinner or birthdays.

After 10-days of sugar detox and following the eating schedule I advised, you'll retrain your palate towards sweet things. Now, you won't crave sugar as much as before and will be able to make better food choices. Things which tasted plain before will taste sweeter to you now.

Some of you might have lost some weight by now, too. Even if not, you'll experience positivity about yourself. Your sleep will be better, your mood will be happier, and your digestive functions will improve and be better than before. What more can you ask for?

So, it's your turn to benefit from the training I have revealed in this book. Training, that's easy, but requires discipline and willpower to get results. Not only will you see physical results, but my training will equip you with the skills and knowledge to ditch your sugar addiction and be in complete control of what you eat.

Do you know the number one benefit of being healthier?

Healthier people are more productive, spend less on healthcare, and have better job securities. They are more active for home and social activities, spend less time in hospitals, doctor offices and pharmacies, have less pain and discomfort, and ultimately live a longer and better quality of life.

So, what are you waiting for?

Take action now! Train your body and mind to live without the added sugars using the advice given in this book, otherwise, you'll miss out on the most productive years of your life.

You don't have to go far to learn these sugar detox tips. You have them right here! Tips and training that are proven to yield results for people of all ages. Whether you are 20 or 40, the tips for detoxing sugar given in this book will prove beneficial for you. All you have to do is ACT ON THEM, NOW!!

The Fastest & Easiest Way To Detox & Eliminate Sugar
In Only 10 Days To Lose Weight And Burn Fat

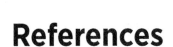

References

-Avena, N. (2007, May 18). *Evidence for sugar addiction: Behavioral and neurochemical effects of intermittent, excessive sugar intake.* PubMed Central (PMC). https://www.ncbi.nlm.nih.gov/pmc/articles/PMC2235907/

What I've Learned. (2016, October 25). *Food Industry's Secret Weapon (WHY Sugar is addictive & in 80% of Food).* YouTube. https://www.youtube.com/watch?v=LPxIssabhTc

Barnwell, A. (2020, January 17). *Secret Sugars: The 56 Different Names for Sugar.* Virta Health. https://www.virtahealth.com/blog/names-for-sugar

After Skool. (2018, June 27). *Cocaine vs Sugar.* YouTube. https://www.youtube.com/watch?v=rrb06DhdrFE&t=10s

The Importance of Developing a Support System. (2014, December 10). BJCEAP. https://www.bjceap.com/Blog/ArtMID/448/ArticleID/139/The-Importance-of-Developing-a-Support-System

Nyorani, C. (n.d.). *4 Simple Strategies to Achieve Your Health Goals.* ThriveGlobal. Retrieved July 8, 2020, from https://thriveglobal.com/stories/4-simple-strategies-to-achieve-your-health-goals/

Pasternak, H. M. (2018, May 31). *Reach Your Fitness Goals by Building a Community of Support.* Oxygen Magazine. https://www.oxygenmag.com/lifestyle/reach-your-fitness-goals-by-building-a-community-of-support

Fight Sugar Addiction by Cleaning Out Your Kitchen. (2016, March 26). Dummies. https://www.dummies.com/health/nutrition/fight-sugar-addiction-by-cleaning-out-your-kitchen/

Hansen, F. (2018, October 29). *Which Fruits Have The Lowest Glycemic Load?* Adrenal Fatigue Solution. https://adrenalfatiguesolution.com/fruits-lowest-glycemic-load/

Types of Nuts and Seeds and Their Health Benefits. (n.d.). Superfoodevolution. Retrieved July 8, 2020, from https://www.superfoodevolution.com/nuts-and-seeds.html

Whitbread, D. (2020, June 27). *Top 10 Beans and Legumes Highest in Protein.* Myfooddata. https://www.myfooddata.com/articles/beans-legumes-highest-protein.php

Tarantino, O. (2019, February 28). *12 Best Sugar-Free Protein Powders.* Eat This Not That. https://www.eatthis.com/unsweetened-protein-powder/

Food, F. (2020, April 10). *Go on a sugar-free diet! Get a list of what to eat and to avoid.* Further Food. https://www.furtherfood.com/going-sugar-free-your-handy-food-guide-of-what-to-eat-what-to-avoid/

Why Soaking Nuts and Seeds is Better for Nutrient Absorption. (n.d.). Superfoodevolution. https://www.superfoodevolution.com/soaking-nuts-and-seeds.html

Levi, A. (2017, October 20). *How to Ease Withdrawal Symptoms When You Quit Sugar, According to a Nutritionist.* Health.Com. https://www.health.com/nutrition/sugar-free-diet-help

Yasin, K. (2054, February 13). *5 No-Sugar Breakfast Recipes.* Healthline. https://www.healthline.com/health/food-nutrition/sugar-free-breakfast-recipes#1.-overnight-oats

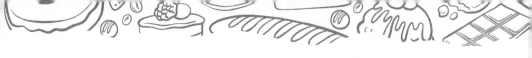

Quick Black Bean Hummus. (2019, July 10). Allrecipes. https://www.allrecipes.com/recipe/240178/quick-black-bean-hummus/

C. (2018, July 11). *This Red Cabbage Salad Is Perfect for a Refreshing Lunch.* Clean Program. https://blog.cleanprogram.com/red-cabbage-salad/#more-6286

Posted By: Meal Prep on Fleek. (2019, December 20). *Sheet Pan Recipe Chicken and Asparagus Bowl.* Meal Prep on FleekTM. https://mealpreponfleek.com/sheet-pan-chicken-asparagus/

Frances. (n.d.). *Pardon Our Interruption.* Oprah.Com. http://www.oprah.com/food/mixed-grain-cereal-with-chai-spice

Guacamole. (2020, February 5). Allrecipes. https://www.allrecipes.com/recipe/14231/guacamole/

Blackened Chicken and Avocado Salad. (2020, July 5). Eatwell101. https://www.eatwell101.com/blackened-chicken-avocado-salad-recipe

Posted By: Meal Prep on Fleek. (2020, May 4). *Sheet Pan Chicken Fajitas.* Meal Prep on FleekTM. https://mealpreponfleek.com/sheet-pan-chicken-fajitas/

Pardon Our Interruption. (n.d.). Oprah.Com. http://www.oprah.com/food/tomato-grits-and-sausage-recipe

Crunchy Sugar-Free Granola. (2018, June 8). Allrecipes. https://www.allrecipes.com/recipe/261939/crunchy-sugar-free-granola/

Posted By: Meal Prep on Fleek. (2020a, May 4). *Carrot Meatballs With Mint Cauliflower Rice.* Meal Prep on FleekTM. https://mealpreponfleek.com/carrot-meatballs-mint-cauliflower-rice/

Posted By: Meal Prep on Fleek. (2020b, May 4). *Sesame Salmon with Baby Bok Choy and Mushrooms*. Meal Prep on FleekTM. https://mealpreponfleek.com/sesame-salmon-baby-bok-choy-mushrooms/

Pardon Our Interruption. (n.d.-b). Oprah.Com. http://www.oprah.com/food/oatmeal-pancakes-recipe

Avocado Banana Green Smoothie | Minimalist Baker Recipes. (2020, May 15). Minimalist Baker. https://minimalistbaker.com/creamy-avocado-banana-green-smoothie/

Posted By: Meal Prep on Fleek. (2020d, May 4). *Skillet Shrimp with Tomato and Avocado*. Meal Prep on FleekTM. https://mealpreponfleek.com/skillet-shrimp-with-tomato-and-avocado/

Posted By: Meal Prep on Fleek. (2020e, May 4). *Spicy Mustard Thyme Chicken & Coconut Roasted Brussels Sprouts*. Meal Prep on FleekTM. https://mealpreponfleek.com/spicy-mustard-thyme-chicken-coconut-roasted-brussels-sprouts/

Gerorgie. (2015, July 13). *STRAWBERRY COCONUT YOGURT BREAKFAST BOWL*. In It 4 the Long Run. http://init4thelongrun.com/2015/07/13/strawberry-coconut-yogurt-breakfast-bowl/

C. (2018b, August 29). *A Watermelon Slushy to Celebrate the End of Summer*. Clean Program. https://blog.cleanprogram.com/watermelon-slushy/#more-6272

C. (2017, July 19). *Summer Salad Brings the Best of the Season*. Clean Program. https://blog.cleanprogram.com/summer-salad/#more-6382

Taste of Home Editors. (n.d.). *Roast Pork with Apples & Onions*. Taste of Home. https://www.tasteofhome.com/recipes/roast-pork-with-apples-onions/

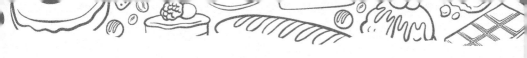

Lederle, D. (2019, April 11). *Mango Coconut Chia Pudding.* The Healthy Maven. https://www.thehealthymaven.com/mango-coconut-chia-pudding

C. (2018c, September 19). *Crunchy Kale Chips Make the Best Snack.* Clean Program. https://blog.cleanprogram.com/kale-chips/

Meal Prep Garlic Butter Chicken Meatballs with Cauliflower Rice. (2020, May 5). Eatwell101. https://www.eatwell101.com/chicken-meatballs-meal-prep-recipe

M. (2020, January 27). *20 Minute Baked Pesto Salmon {Low Carb, Whole30, Paleo}.* Skinny Fitalicious. https://skinnyfitalicious.com/baked-pesto-salmon/

Layla. (n.d.-b). *Healthy 2 Ingredient Pancakes (Paleo, Gluten & Dairy-Free, No Sugar added.* Gimme Delicious. https://gimmedelicious.com/healthy-2-ingredient-paleo-pancakes-gluten-dairy-free-no-sugar-added/

Meal, E. T. S. K. |. (2019, September 11). *Best Steak Salad with Creamy Balsamic Vinaigrette.* The Endless Meal®. https://www.theendlessmeal.com/best-steak-salad/

Taste of Home Editors. (n.d.-a). *Deviled Chicken.* Taste of Home. https://www.tasteofhome.com/recipes/deviled-chicken/

M. (2019, July 25). *Almond Butter Blueberry Paleo Waffles.* Ambitious Kitchen. https://www.ambitiouskitchen.com/almond-butter-blueberry-paleo-waffles/

C. (2019a, October 25). *Lavender Blueberry Smoothie with Cauliflower (And It's Actually Good).* Clean Program. https://blog.cleanprogram.com/blueberry-smoothie/

Kim. (2019b, October 14). *CREAMY GARLIC MUSHROOM CHICKEN.* My Sugar Free Kitchen. https://www.mysugarfreekitchen.com/creamy-garlic-mushroom-chicken/

A. (2019a, June 24). *Cajun Shrimp and Rice.* Everyday Easy Eats. https://www.everydayeasyeats.com/cajun-shrimp-and-rice-recipe/

J. (2020a, March 20). *Breakfast Fried Brown Rice.* How Sweet Eats. https://www.howsweeteats.com/2015/06/breakfast-fried-rice/

C. (2017a, March 8). *Beet Hummus: Your Surprising New Favorite.* Clean Program. https://blog.cleanprogram.com/beet-hummus/

Ford, S. (2019, July 10). *Kale, Quinoa, and Avocado Salad with Lemon Dijon Vinaigrette.* Allrecipes. https://www.allrecipes.com/recipe/230050/kale-quinoa-and-avocado-salad-with-lemon-dijon-vinaigrette/

Taste of Home Editors. (n.d.-b). *Grilled Basil Chicken and Tomatoes.* Taste of Home. https://www.tasteofhome.com/recipes/grilled-basil-chicken-and-tomatoes/

C. (2018a, May 2). T*his Gluten-Free Avocado Toast Has a Special Ingredient.* Clean Program. https://blog.cleanprogram.com/avocado-toast/#more-6305

Coconut and Mandarin Orange Vegan Smoothie Bowl. (2016, December 23). Amy Gorin Nutrition. https://www.amydgorin.com/vegan-mandarin-orange-creamy-coconut-smoothie-bowl/

Garlic Ginger Shrimp Meal Prep with Quinoa and Tomato Salsa. (2020, May 9). Eatwell101. https://www.eatwell101.com/shrimp-meal-prep-recipe

Taste of Home Editors. (n.d.-a). *Cumin-Chili Spiced Flank Steak.* Taste of Home. https://www.tasteofhome.com/recipes/cumin-chili-spiced-flank-steak/

Mattison, L. D. (2018, July 3). *How to Make Homemade Hot Sauce.* Taste of Home. https://www.tasteofhome.com/article/how-to-make-homemade-hot-sauce/

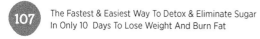

C. (2018a, April 18). *How to Make an Easy Kimchi.* Clean Program. https://blog.cleanprogram.com/kimchi/

Lindsay. (2019, January 15). *Our Life Without Sugar.* Pinch of Yum. https://pinchofyum.com/our-life-without-sugar

Whelan, C. (749, January 10). *No-Sugar Diet: 10 Tips to Get Started.* Healthline. https://www.healthline.com/health/food-nutrition/no-sugar-diet#takeaway

Diane. (n.d.-a). *WHAT SHOULD I DO AFTER THE 21-DAY SUGAR DETOX?* The 21 Day Sugar Detox. https://21daysugardetox.com/what-should-i-do-after-the-21-day-sugar-detox/

Dr Brent Baldasare. (2017, March 13). *Sugar vs Cocaine.* YouTube. https://www.youtube.com/watch?v=bKG1JNq7RyM

McKay, T. (2014, April 21). *What Happens to Your Brain on Sugar, Explained by Science.* Mic. https://www.mic.com/articles/88015/what-happens-to-your-brain-on-sugar-explained-by-science

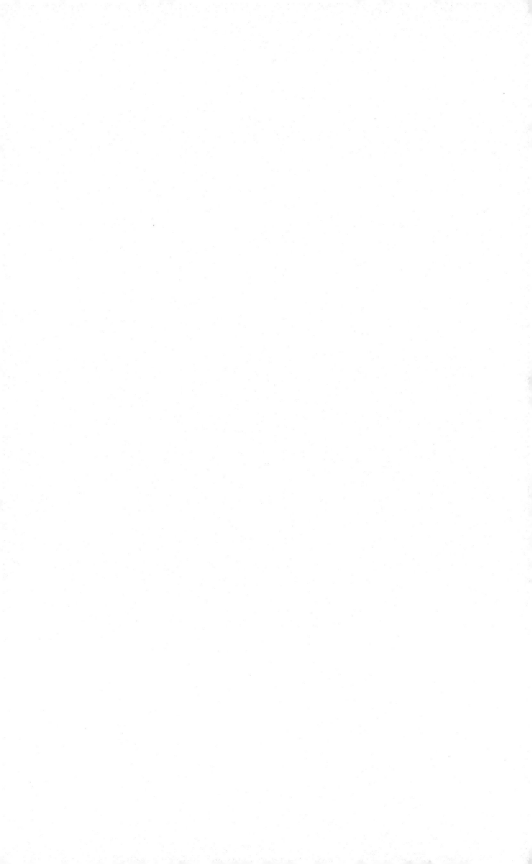

Printed in Great Britain
by Amazon